Instructor's Manual to Accompany

PSYCHIATRIC MENTAL HEALTH NURSING

2nd EDITION

UNDERSTANDING THE CLIENT AS WELL AS THE CONDITION

Instructor's Manual to Accompany

PSYCHIATRIC MENTAL HEALTH NURSING

2nd EDITION

UNDERSTANDING THE CLIENT AS WELL AS THE CONDITION

Noreen Cavan Frisch, RN, PhD, FAAN
Professor and Chair
Department of Nursing
Cleveland State University
Cleveland, Ohio

And

Lawrence E. Frisch, MPH, PhD
Department of Preventive Medicine
The University of Kansas School of Medicine—Wichita
Wichita, Kansas

Instructor's Manual
Prepared by

Brenda P. Johnson, RN, PhD
Assistant Professor
Department of Nursing
Southeast Missouri State University
Cape Girardeau, Missouri

DELMAR
THOMSON LEARNING™

Australia Canada Mexico Singapore Spain United Kingdom United States

DELMAR
THOMSON LEARNING™

NOTICE TO THE READER

Publisher does not warrant or guarantee any of the products described herein or perform any independent analysis in connection with any of the product information contained herein. Publisher does not assume, and expressly disclaims, any obligation to obtain and include information other than that provided to it by the manufacturer.

The reader is expressly warned to consider and adopt all safety precautions that might be indicated by the activities herein and to avoid all potential hazards. By following the instructions contained herein, the reader willingly assumes all risks in connection with such instructions.

The Publisher makes no representation or warranties of any kind, including but not limited to, the warranties of fitness for particular purpose or merchantability, nor are any such representations implied with respect to the material set forth herein, and the publisher takes no responsibility with respect to such material. The publisher shall not be liable for any special, consequential, or exemplary damages resulting, in whole or part, from the readers' use of, or reliance upon, this material.

Delmar Staff
Health Care Publishing Director: William Brottmiller
Executive Marketing Manager: Dawn F. Gerrain
Executive Editor: Cathy L. Esperti
Acquisitions Editor: Matthew Kane
Developmental Editor: Marjorie A. Bruce
Editorial Assistant: Shelley Esposito
Project Editor: Maureen M.E. Grealish
Production Coordinator: Nina Lontrato/Sherry McGaughan
Art/Design Coordinator: Robert Plante

Printed in the United States of America
3 4 5 XXX 05 04 03 02

For more information, contact Delmar Learning, Executive Woods, 5 Maxwell Drive, Clifton Park, NY 12065
World Wide Web at http://www.delmar.com

ISBN: 0-7668-4173-1

Psychiatric Mental Health Nursing 2nd Edition
By Noreen Cavan Frisch and Lawrence E. Frisch
Prepared by Brenda P. Johnson

Contents

Unit

1

Foundations for Practice

The nine chapters of Unit I provide the foundational materials for psychiatric mental health nursing (PMHN). The content of these chapters includes philosophical, historical, theoretical, cultural, ethical, legal, and epidemiological information. Specific diagnostic elements for PMHN are delineated. The nursing process, the nurse-client relationship, and the communication process are reviewed.

The chapters of Unit I provide the foundation for grounded practice in the psychiatric mental health arena. From this foundation, the student can better understand the content on clinical disorders, the needs of special populations, and treatment modalities.

NOTES

Through the Door: Your First Day in Psychiatric Nursing

Chapter 1

Competencies

Upon completion of this chapter the learner will be able to:

1. Reflect on the experience of a psychiatric nursing course as a rite of passage in the process of becoming a nurse.
2. Describe basic information about the nature and practice of psychiatric mental health care, including
   - The nature of mental health and mental illness
   - A sense of why a person is hospitalized for psychiatric care
   - Basic job descriptions and education of various mental health workers
   - Concerns and advice from prior students
3. Interpret the goal of psychiatric care as that of strengthening the healthy portion of the client.

Key Terms

Depression	Hallucination	Mental health
Disability	Mania	Mental illness
Distress	Mental disorder	Psychosis

Teaching Methods and Strategies

This chapter sets the tone for learning experiences in psychiatric mental health nursing. It leads the student through the door to critical thinking about mental health and mental illness, and frames the experience as a rite of passage for one's nursing career. As such, teaching methods that foster self-reflection and discussion are suggested. In addition, selected self-disclosure about the educator's journey through psychiatric nursing is appropriate. These exchanges need to be tempered by the realization that, for most students, this is a time of fear, growth, and transformation.

The author has provided several reflective thinking boxes in this chapter that lend themselves to individual assignments and group discussions. Several suggested assignments appear in the learning activities section. Reflective thinking questions provide a base for the development of critical thinking. Critical thinking entails purposeful, goal-directed consideration of facts and principles using the scientific method. It involves making judgments based on evidence versus assumptions. In so doing, strategies can be developed to maximize the individual's potential and solve problems.

Often the "answers" stimulate even more questions. This process of questioning, investigating, and re-examining builds the critical thinking abilities of the student, which are so important to moving from novice to competent, practicing nurse. In the psychiatric care setting, the questions often involve self-reflection, examining one's values, and uncovering assumptions that underscore how the person engages life. This growth-producing process is also very personal. For this reason, many critical thinking exercises are best suited for small group discussion versus classroom setting application.

The actual process of critical thinking has several interdependent elements. The educator needs to clearly identify the purpose or goal and the problem to be resolved or the questions at issue. Different points of view are illuminated and discussed in view of evidence and past experience. The assumptions and key concepts, which are implicit in the person's thinking, are made explicit so they are examined for accuracy and applicability to the given situation. From this perspective, inferences, implications, and consequences can be examined.

Chapter 1 is the logical place to introduce students to the strategy of using a journal to write an ongoing account of the experiential process of transformation through psychiatric nursing and critical thinking. The faculty has the role of facilitator and encourager to enable the student to honestly explore the experiences. Often students believe they must record only socially approved, expectation-driven comments so the educator is challenged to create an environment in which the student can openly share experiences.

Lesson Plans

Topic: Introduction to the Experience of Psychiatric Mental Health Nursing

Competency 1.1

Reflect on the notion of the psychiatric mental health nursing course as a rite of passage.

CONTENT OUTLINE

- Define the phrase *rite of passage.*
- Describe the elements of role transformation.
- Describe the expectations related to psychiatric mental health nursing.

METHOD

Lecture
Discussion
Reflective thinking exercise

Competency 1.2a

Describe the continuum of mental health and mental illness.

CONTENT OUTLINE

- Define mental health.
- Define mental illness.
- Define distress.
- Describe the notion of degrees of dysfunction.

METHOD

Lecture
Discussion
Slide/transparency
Reflective thinking exercise

Competency 1.2b

Describe the reasons a person is hospitalized for psychiatric care.

CONTENT OUTLINE

- Define the terms *normal* and *mental illness.*
- Define the terms *psychosis, depression, mania, hallucinations, delusions,* and *normal.*
- Review these terms with respect to the continuum of mental health and mental illness.
- Describe the concept of inability for self-care.
- Describe the concept of threat to self or others.
- Review the boxed information: Signs of Mental Illness.

METHOD

Lecture
Discussion
Slides/transparencies
Discussion of the excerpt "Parallel Universe"

Competency 1.2c

Compare and contrast the roles and educational requirements of various mental health workers.

CONTENT OUTLINE

- Review Table 1-1: Mental Health Professionals.
- Describe the two levels of psychiatric nursing practice.

METHOD

Lecture
Slide/transparency

Competency 1.2d

Discuss the typical concerns and advice of students who have already completed an educational experience in psychiatric mental health nursing.

CONTENT OUTLINE

- Identify one concern of students who have completed their education in mental health nursing.
- List other concerns identified by prior students.
- Identify strategies to cope with fears.
- Review tips for conversing with mentally ill persons.
- Identify other resources to assist students to deal with concerns.

METHOD

Lecture
Discussion
Slide/transparency
Reflective thinking exercise
Role play

Competency 1.3

Describe the goal of: (1) psychiatric mental health care; (2) psychiatric mental health nursing educational experience.

CONTENT OUTLINE

- Describe the concept of use of "self."
- Discuss the emphasis on communication.
- Review the importance of self-reflection to personal and professional development.

METHOD

Discussion
Role play

Learning Experiences

Theory Application

IN THE BEGINNING

• It is suggested that the first class be initiated by asking the questions in the opening box and the reflective thinking section of this chapter.

1. What have been your experiences with and exposure to psychiatric care?
2. What are your ideas and images of psychiatry and mental health care?
3. What are your feelings about taking a course in psychiatric mental health nursing?
4. What do you expect to see on a psychiatric unit or in a community psychiatric care agency?

Individual Activities

JOURNALING

• Instruct students to keep an ongoing record of their experiences during the psychiatric mental health course. The focus is on the experience, in the personal sense, which is the essence of the transformational rite of passage associated with this clinical area. Have students begin by defining mental illness and mental health in their own words.

EXPECTATIONS

• Assign students the task of answering the questions listed below. In class, request student volunteers to share some of their responses.

1. What do you think this clinical experience will be like?
2. In two sentences, how would you describe mental illness?
3. In two sentences, how would you describe mental health?
4. What do you think you will be doing during the course in psychiatric mental health nursing?

Group Activities

DISCUSSION OF CONCERNS

• Distribute a 3 × 5 card to each student in the class. Then divide the class into small groups (four to six students per group). Instruct each group to select a reporter. Next, instruct the students to print *one* concern about psychiatric mental health experience on the card and to pass them to the reporter. Within the small group, instruct students to discuss the concerns on the cards, as read by the reporter, so that anonymity can be maintained. After 10 minutes, ask the reporters to share the compiled group list with the class. Open discussion of similar responses is suggested. Finally, the faculty discusses possible methods to deal with the list of concerns.

DEFINITIONS OF MENTAL HEALTH AND MENTAL ILLNESS

1. In small groups, ask each student to discuss his or her own definitions of mental illness and mental health. When they have finished sharing their individual perspectives, ask them to synthesize the information into a "group" definition of mental health and mental illness. Ask for a volunteer from each group to read the final products to the class.
2. In addition to the process described in part 1, distribute a sheet of newsprint or poster paper to each small group. Have them record the synthesized "group" definitions on the paper. Ask each group to post the recorded definitions on the wall and then read all responses to the class. Discuss the similarities, differences, and any misconceptions with the class.

Clinical Activities

ROLES OF MENTAL HEALTH CARE WORKERS

• Assign each student to interview a nurse and one other health care worker. The faculty will assign a member of the health care team (physician, psychologist, social worker, activity therapist, pharmacist, mental health tech, or other). Each person interviewed is asked the following:

1. Define mental health.
2. Define mental illness.
3. Describe your role in the delivery of care to psychiatric clients.

The responses are then shared in clinical conference.

THERAPEUTIC USE OF SELF

• After the first day's experiences in the psychiatric mental health area, discuss with students their individual perspectives on therapeutic use of self. Highlight the skills involved in therapeutic use of self, including (but not limited to) communication, presence, listening, appropriate disclosure, and advocacy.

Internet Activities

- McLean Hospital is still in operation and has a web site: http://www.mcleanhospital.org
- Visit the site for the National Institute of Mental Health: http://www.nimh.nih.gov

NOTES

Psychiatric Nursing: The Evolution of a Specialty

Chapter 2

Competencies

Upon completion of this chapter, the learner will be able to:

1. Describe changes in societal attitudes toward mental illness leading to the identification of mental illness as a disease.
2. Discuss the medicalization of mental illness in the 18th and 19th centuries.
3. Explain why nurses working with the mentally ill in the 19th century did not identify with nurses providing physical care.
4. Identify factors that brought nursing of the physically ill and nursing of the mentally ill together.
5. Describe the role of psychiatric nursing today as a core subject and content area of nursing practice.
6. Identify the evolving role of psychiatric nursing in community settings.

Key Terms

Asylum
Brown Report
National Mental Health Act
Psychiatric mental health advanced practice registered nurse
Psychiatric mental health nurse

Teaching Methods and Strategies

This chapter is designed to provide the historical perspective for the evolution of the current practice of psychiatric mental health nursing. The information in this chapter contains a number of historical facts. Developing interesting methods to bring history to life requires the educator to draw on a variety of methods. Depending on the creative tendencies of the individual(s) doing the instruction, teaching methods may include word games, picture associations, role playing, and simulation of a debate among several of the historical figures to portray their respective perspectives. The major constraint is consideration of how much teaching time can be devoted to this historical information. Faculty may opt for limiting the time commitment to this information to ensure adequate time to teach other application- and practice-based content. Throughout the chapter the most important historical information has been pulled together into tables and boxed areas.

The reflective thinking questions in Chapter 2 provide the educator with the threads to stimulate discussion about the notion of normalcy, deviance, and how societies deal with deviation. When these questions are used to examine the historical changes in the care of the mentally ill, the student can better understand how society defines health, illness, and the notion of a need to provide care. The philosophical perspectives and key players in the evolution of compassionate care provided by trained and educated individuals through the 18th and 19th centuries are succinctly presented. This information lends itself to role playing as well as learning through printed materials.

Tables in this chapter highlight the salient historical elements that formed the foundations for the evolution of psychiatric mental health nursing (PMHN) as a specialty. Table 2-1 provides an overview of the early theories that led to the emergence of nursing education and nursing care of the mentally ill. These are only peripheral to the historical events in psychiatric nursing history that are summarized in Table 2-2.

The guidelines for current PMHN practice are summarized in boxed information from the American Nurses Association Standards of Psychiatric Mental Health Nursing Practice and the Statement of Psychiatric Mental Health Nursing Practice. The specifics of the areas of practice for PMHN, its "phenomena of concern" and levels of certification are described. A summary of community-based roles in PMHN is also provided in boxed format with notes about additional information found in other chapters of the text.

The educator may wish to vivify these descriptions by inviting a panel of nurses with different levels of preparation who practice in a variety of locations and settings to present to the class. To facilitate a more active participative approach, students can be assigned to interview a nurse working in the psychiatric area, a nurse certified in PMHN, and a nurse with certification as an advanced practice PMHN.

Lesson Plans

Topic: Evolution of the Psychiatric Nursing Specialty

Competency 2.1

Describe societal changes in attitudes toward mental illness leading to the identification of mental illness as a disease.

CONTENT OUTLINE

- Identify historical views of causes and treatment for mental illness held during different periods: early civilizations, Middle Ages, and Renaissance:
  - Demonic possession
  - Breaking taboo
  - Effect of harmful substance
  - Body humors
  - Influence of the moon
- Describe the treatment of the mentally ill in the early periods of civilization:
  - Magic
  - Prayer
  - Seclusion
  - Incarceration
  - Punishment
  - Care provided by untrained persons

METHOD

Lecture
Audio visual

Competency 2.2

Discuss the medicalization of mental illness in the 18th and 19th centuries.

CONTENT OUTLINE

- Describe the changes in care initiated by Dr. William Battie in England.
- Discuss the shift in focus from character disorder to disease.
- Describe the various theories of causation associated with the notion of mental illness as a disease process.
- Discuss the strengths and limitations of "asylums" for the treatment of the insane.

METHOD

Lecture
Small group discussion

Competency 2.3

Explain why nurses working with the mentally ill in the 19th century did not identify with nurses providing physical care.

CONTENT OUTLINE

- Describe the evolution of the nurse's role in the care of the mentally ill:
  - Moving from unskilled caretaker to skilled caregiver to educated care provider
  - Moving from guard to compassionate attendant
  - Schools for mental health nurses as separate from other nursing education: McLean Training School (medical model vs. Nightingale model of autonomous nursing training)

METHOD

Lecture
Photographic illustrations

Competency 2.4

Identify factors that brought nursing of the physically ill and nursing of the mentally ill together.

CONTENT OUTLINE

- Discuss changes in the nursing care arena beginning at the 1893 World's Fair conference:
  - Call for clear standards for nursing education and definition of "trained nurse"
  - Skills for mental health nurses included those for physical and mental care (custodial care, supervision of ward attendants, cold dressings, poltices, wet wraps, baths, drugs for violent clients)
- Identify the late 19th century nursing reform leaders Isabel Hampton and Lavinia Dock.
- Describe the 20th century changes in mental health nursing:
  - *1907* American Psychiatric Association report on standards for mental nursing care (physician control)
  - *1913* Johns Hopkins Hospital School included training in psychiatric care for all nurses
  - *1920* Publication of first psychiatric nursing textbook
  - *1937* National League for Nursing (NLN) recommendation for psychiatric nursing as part of all nursing education
  - *1946* National Mental Health Act to establish funding and graduate education
  - *1948* Brown Report "The Future of Nursing"
  - *1952* Publication of "Interpersonal Relations in Nursing"
  - *1955* NLN requirement for clinical experience as well as classroom information on psychiatric nursing
  - *1961* Publication of "The Dynamic Nurse Patient Relationship"
  - *1960s* Journals established: *Perspectives in Psychiatric Care* and *Journal of Psychiatric (Psychosocial) Nursing and Mental Health Services*
- Identify 20th century nursing leaders: Effie Taylor, Harriet Bailey, Ester Lucille Brown, Hildegard Peplau, and Ida Jeane Orlando.

METHOD

Lecture
Slide/transparency

Competency 2.5

Describe the role of psychiatric nursing today as a core subject and content area of nursing practice.

CONTENT OUTLINE

- Define psychiatric nursing as per American Nurses Association (ANA) standards.
- Discuss the levels of psychiatric nursing practice delineated in the ANA 1994 Standards of Psychiatric Mental Health Clinical Nursing Practice:

  Basic level: Registered nurse, baccalaureate education, clinically skilled; educate, promote health, assess dysfunction, regain/improve coping

  Advanced level (Advanced Practice Registered Nurse, or APRN): Licensed registered nurse, graduate education, clinical specialist; range of activities, psychotherapy, and consultation
- Describe the relationship of research and theory development to the practice of psychiatric mental health nursing.

METHOD

Lecture
Slide/transparency

Competency 2.6

Identify the evolving role of psychiatric nursing in community settings.

CONTENT OUTLINE

- Highlight the influences of socioeconomic factors on the delivery of care, especially managed care.
- Describe the shift in settings to the community:

  Home health care
  School-based centers
  Mobile treatment units
  Community-based behavioral care centers

METHOD

Lecture

Learning Experiences

Theory Application

• Presenting historical information in a manner that revivifies the experiences within the context of the era helps students better understand the evolution of the role of the psychiatric mental health nurse. Drawing a parallel between a given era and the medical/nursing practice at the time can be used later to present information about the development of different clinical diagnostic criteria, regulations and acts, and treatment modalities.

Individual Activities

• Assign students to write a paragraph about what they perceive to be the current status of care for the mentally ill. Have them date the paragraph, seal it in an envelope, and keep it in their journal until the last day of the experience. Then, review it and note how their perceptions have changed since the first week of class.

Group Activities

• Discussion: What is the current state of care for the mentally ill?

Have students anonymously turn in a copy of the paragraph written about their perception of the care for the mentally ill. Redistribute the papers randomly. Ask a volunteer to begin the discussion by reading the paragraph to the group. Instruct any students who have similar paragraphs to share any additional information. Then ask students to share paragraphs that have differing perspectives. Open the discussion to other perceptions. Summarize and clarify as appropriate.

• Debate: The Asylum Model of Care

Divide the students into three groups: audience, pro team (up to five members) and con team (up to five members). One team is to provide the arguments pro asylum care while the other team presents the con viewpoint. The role of the audience is to listen to the debate. The faculty member serves as the moderator.

First each team takes no more than 3 minutes to present its salient points. This is followed by 5 minutes for rebuttal by each team. Finally, each team presents closing points (2 minutes). After the presentation, a vote is taken among the participant group: yea or nay the asylum model. This is followed by open discussion among all members of the student group.

• Discussion Group: What is the impact of managed care on mental health practice?

Assign students to read at least one article about managed care and behavioral health care practice as the basis for the discussion. Then have students voice their own opinions about the current state of health care for the mentally ill.

Clinical Activities

• Instruct students to interview the members of the psychiatric nursing staff who represent the "newest" psychiatric nurse and the "most seasoned" psychiatric nurse. Ask each nurse to describe her ideas about care for the mentally ill from when she started to the present time. Then ask each nurse for the three things that she believes make the most difference in caring for the mentally ill.

Internet Activities

• Link to the site for the American Psychiatric Nurses Association: http://www.apna.org

NOTES

Theory as Basis for Practice

Chapter 3

Competencies

Upon completion of this chapter, the learner will be able to:

1. Discuss the relationship between practice, theory, and research.
2. Define terminology related to theory.
3. Identify the major components of selected nursing theories.
4. Discuss psychosocial theories from other disciplines useful in psychiatric nursing practice.
5. Consider various theories as a guide to nursing practice.

Key Terms

Adaptive potential
Cognition
Concept
Conceptual framework
Created environment
Cultural care
Cultural care accommodation/negotiation
Cultural care preservation/maintenance
Cultural care repatterning/restructuring
Culture
Ego
External environment
Extrapersonal stressor
Fixation
Folk system
Id
Internal environment
Interpersonal stressor
Intrapersonal stressor
Modeling
Nursing agency
Nursing situation
Professional system
Regression
Role modeling
Self-care
Self-care agency
Self-care deficit
Superego
Theory
Therapeutic self-care demand

Teaching Methods and Strategies

Nursing is a discipline in which practice is derived from theory and where theories have been tested by research. The relationship between theory, practice, and research is continuously intertwined in professional nursing.

Chapter 3 provides the theoretical basis for understanding the complex intricacies of psychiatric mental health nursing practice. The content of this chapter will establish the foundation for understanding information presented in later chapters of the textbook. The information in this chapter can be considered an overview or survey of a broad range of theories. In addition, many key terms used throughout the psychiatric nursing experience are explained in this chapter.

The wise educator will devote time to teaching and reviewing the theoretical information and carefully reflect on the specific learning needs of the student cohort. Some students may be well versed in nursing theory while others have a working knowledge of psychological theories. Still others will have little background information and must rely on the educator to build the foundation.

Teaching about theories can be approached from several perspectives. If a mastery perspective is taken, elements of the theory, important names and dates, key concepts, and principles can be presented with a goal of memorization. A more dynamic perspective takes the basic information laid out in the mastery approach and vivifies the information with a variety of examples and discussion applied to clinical situations. A third approach is to integrate the elements of different theories throughout the full range of content presented in the textbook. The choice of approach depends on the experiential background of the student and the faculty.

Lesson Plans

Topic: Theory as a Basis for Practice

Competency 3.1

Discuss the relationship between practice, theory, and research.

CONTENT OUTLINE

- Describe the delivery of care (practice) as built around theoretical frameworks derived from tested/researched theories.

METHOD

Lecture
Slide/transparency
Reflective thinking exercise
Case example

Competency 3.2

Define terminology related to theory.

CONTENT OUTLINE

- Define the key terms *concept, conceptual framework,* and *theory.*
- Define the term *nursing theory.*

METHOD

Lecture

Competency 3.3

Identify the major components of selected nursing theories.

CONTENT OUTLINE

- Discuss the nursing theories that focus on relationships (Hildegard Peplau, Helen Erickson et al.).
- Describe the focus, major concepts, and operating principles of each theoretical framework:

  Peplau Focus of Interpersonal Nursing theory is the therapeutic interpersonal relationship. Components include nurse, client, professional expertise, client need. Phases of the interpersonal relationship are orientation, identification, exploitation, and resolution.

  Erickson et al. Focus of Modeling theory is on interpersonal interactive skills for role enactment. Major concepts include: modeling, role modeling, aims of intervention (to promote trust, positive orientation, perceived control, strengths, and health-directed mutual goals), self-care (knowledge, resources, and action), affiliative-individuation, and adaptive potential. Modeling involves assessment and understanding of the client's perception of the world and role modeling involves development of care based on the client's worldview. Five principles:

  1. A trusting and functional nurse-client relationship exists.
  2. Affiliative-individuation is dependent on client's perception of self as acceptable, respectable, and worthwhile.
  3. Human development depends on a perception of control over one's life.
  4. There is an innate drive for holistic health.
  5. Human growth is dependent on satisfaction of basic needs.

- Discuss the nursing theories that focus on the concept of caring (Jean Watson, Madeleine Leininger, and Anne Boykin and Savina Schoenhofer).
- Describe the focus, major concepts, and operating principles of each theoretical framework:

  Watson Focus of the Science of Caring theory is on caring as the domain of nursing. Assumptions about the science of nursing:

  1. Effective caring is based on interpersonal relationship.
  2. Caring includes carative factors.
  3. Carative factors lead to satisfying human needs and promoting growth and health.
  4. The person is accepted now and in the future.
  5. Potential is developed while supporting personal choice.
  6. Caring is healthogenic and integrative.
  7. Caring is central to nursing.

  Theoretical framework based on ten carative factors and the first three factors form the foundation for the other seven factors:

  1. Humanistic-altruistic system of values
  2. Instillation of hope
  3. Cultivation of sensitivity
  4. Development of a helping and trusting relationship
  5. Promotion and acceptance of feelings (positive and negative)
  6. Use of scientific problem solving for decision making
  7. Promotion of interpersonal teaching-learning
  8. Provision for a supportive, protective, and/or corrective environment (physical, mental, sociocultural, and spiritual)
  9. Assistance with gratification of human needs
  10. Allowance for existential-phenomenological forces

  Leininger Focus of Cultural Care Diversity and Universality theory is on culturally congruent care resulting from nursing decisions and actions that are structured as cultural preservation, accommodation, or repatterning. Leininger believes that understanding a specific culture's technology, religion, philosophy, kinship and social relationships, politics, law, economics, and education will contribute to a nurse's knowledge of an individual client and her needs. Major concepts include: culture (learned and shared values, beliefs, norms, and lifeways that guide thinking and actions of a group), cultural care, folk systems, professional systems, nursing and professional nursing, cultural care preservation/maintenance, cultural care accommodation/negotiation, and cultural care repatterning/restructuring.

  Boykin & Schoenhofer Focus of the grand theory of Living Caring theory is that nursing is caring, a process of living caring in the context of relationships and responsibilities for self and others associated with these relationships. It is based on the premise that all persons are caring, but not all acts are caring acts. Seven assumptions:

1. Persons are caring by virtue of their humanness.
2. Caring occurs moment to moment.
3. Caring is whole and complete in the moment.
4. Personhood is a process of living in caring.
5. Personhood is enhanced in nurturing relationships with caring others.
6. Nursing is both discipline and profession.
7. Persons are viewed as already complete, unfolding caring possibilities moment to moment.

- Discuss the nursing theories that focus on the concept of energy fields (Martha Rogers, Rosemarie Parse, and Margaret Newman).
- Describe the focus, major concepts, and operating principles of each theoretical framework:

Rogers Focus is on the science of unitary human beings. Five assumptions about human beings are that:

1. Humans are unified wholes and indivisible.
2. There is a constant exchange of energy and matter between humans and their environments.
3. The life process of human beings evolves irreversibly and unidirectionally.
4. Wholeness of humans is reflected in their patterns.
5. Humans are capable of imagery, thought, abstraction, language, sensation, and emotion.

Major concepts are energy fields, openness, pattern, and pandimensionality. Principles of homeodynamics are integrality, resonancy, and helicy. Health is defined by each individual as a personal value.

Parse Focus is on the existential phenomenological perspective of human becoming. Assumptions about humans include that human beings are:

1. Co-existing in rhythmic patterns with the universe
2. Open beings of free choice and responsibility for decisions
3. Living unities continuously relating
4. Transcending multidimensionality

Assumptions about becoming: Becoming is

1. An open process experienced by the human
2. A rhythmic human-universe process
3. The human's pattern of relating value priorities
4. An intersubjective process of transcending
5. Human evolving

Assumptions about human becoming: Human becoming is

1. Freely choosing personal meaning in the intersubjective process of relating value priorities
2. Co-creating rhythmic patterns of relating in an open process with the universe
3. Co-transcending multidimensionality with emerging possibilities

Themes of human becoming are meaning, rhythmicity, and co-transcendence. Key concepts of structuring meaning are imaging, valuing, and languaging. Key concepts of living the paradoxical unity of patterns of relating are that they can be revealing-concealing, enabling-limiting, and connecting-separating. Key concepts of co-transcending possibilities include powering, originating, and transforming.

Newman Focus is on the concept of health as expanding consciousness and nursing as a unitary-transforming paradigm. Key concepts include movement, time, and space; consciousness, expanding consciousness, pattern, and pattern recognition; transformation and choice point. Health and disease are a meaningful reflection of the whole, shifting to searching for patterns and information about patterns versus symptoms and negative disease states.

- Discuss the nursing theories that focus on when nursing care is needed (Dorothea Orem, Callista Roy, and Betty Neuman).
- Describe the focus, major concepts, and operating principles of each theoretical framework:

Orem Focus of Self-Care Deficit theory is on the interrelated theories of self-care, self-care deficit, and nursing systems. Central concepts include self-care, self-care requisites (universal and developmental), self-care agency, therapeutic self-care demand, self-care deficit, nursing agency, nursing system, and basic conditioning factors. The nursing system is defined by the type of self-care deficit, and may be wholly compensatory, partially compensatory, supportive-educative, or supportive-developmental.

Roy Focus on the Adaptation model where the person processes environmental stimuli through coping mechanisms and the goal of nursing is to promote adaptive responses. Essential elements are the person or system, environment, health, and nursing. Coping mechanisms include the cognator subsystem processes and the regulator subsystem processes. Four adaptive modes are physiological, self-concept, role function, and interdependence. Six steps in the adaptive nursing process are:

1. First-level assessment
2. Second-level assessment
3. Nursing diagnosis
4. Goal setting

5. Intervention
6. Evaluation

Neuman Focus of the Neuman Systems model is on the person's reaction to stress, using general systems theory as a basis for application to nursing. The goal of all systems is to achieve optimal stability through the dynamic, repeating cycles of input, throughput, output, and feedback with the environment. The central core of the system represents basic survival factors centered on the physiological, psychological, sociocultural, developmental, and spiritual variables. Key concepts include: lines of resistance, normal line of defense, flexible line of defense, environment, and stressors. System environment may be described in terms of the internal environment, external environment, and created environment. Interventions are grouped as primary, secondary, or tertiary prevention.

METHOD

Discussion of the application of nursing theories presented in Tables 3-1 through 3-4
Slide/transparency
Didactic presentation

Competency 3.4

Discuss psychosocial theories from other disciplines useful in psychiatric nursing practice.

CONTENT OUTLINE

- Describe the psychoanalytical theoretical perspectives of Sigmund Freud, Erik Erikson, and Harry S. Sullivan.
- Describe the focus, major concepts, and operating principles of psychoanalytical theory:

Freud Known for his delineation of the personality as id, ego, and superego and for the related stages of psychosexual development. Id is impulse driven to maximize pleasure and minimize pain. Ego serves to delay immediate impulse gratification, bringing reality into consideration. Superego inhibits impulses that are deemed "wrong," sometimes called the conscience. Psychosexual stages of development occur in sequence and the energy is focused on specific zones or regions of the body:

- *Oral stage* (birth–1 and a half years): Pleasure is associated with mouth and feeding.
- *Anal stage* (1 and a half–3 years): Child is aware of pleasurable sensations associated with bowel movement. Involves the first request of others for child to renounce the instinctual impulse for toilet training.
- *Phallic stage* (3–6 years): Interested in genitalia; parent of opposite sex is desired; same sex parent is seen as rival. These conflicting feelings lead to a variety of defense mechanisms, especially repression and identification, or development of Oedipal (boy) or Electra (girl) complex when unresolved.
- *Latency stage* (6–11 years): When superego and its associated defense mechanisms develop. Sexual feelings and memories from previous three stages are repressed and energies are directed toward socially acceptable activities.
- *Puberty* (11–18 years): Related to independence from parents and finding own mate.

Associated concepts of psychosexual development include fixation and regression.

Erikson Expanded on Freud's theories and identified eight stages of development with a specific ego crisis to be faced during each stage. Biological maturation and social forces compel the individual to move through all stages whether or not the crisis has been successfully resolved:

- *Trust vs. mistrust* (birth–1 and a half years): Development of ego strength to delay gratification.
- *Autonomy vs. shame and doubt* (1 and a half years–3 years): Exercising choice and self-determination.
- *Initiative vs. guilt* (3–6 years): Exploration and discovery as well as discovery of social taboos that lead to guilt.
- *Industry vs. inferiority* (6–11 years): This is the time of adolescence with profound energy, dramatic physiological changes, and new social conflicts. The person is self-absorbed and searching for who one is with the challenge for integration (identity).
- *Identity vs. role confusion* (11–20 years): A period of development of one's personal identity.
- *Intimacy vs. isolation* (18–25 years): The task of young adulthood is to develop enough of a sense of identity to mutually relate to another in an intimate manner.
- *Generativity vs. stagnation* (21–45 years): The person looks beyond self to productivity via work and creation and care of children.
- *Ego integrity vs. despair* (45 years–death): A period of growth, wisdom, and acceptance.

Sullivan Emphasis is on the importance of interpersonal relationships in a more holistic manner. Three life processes: genetic organization, communal existence, and functional activity. Development is influenced by interpersonal relationships experienced: infancy, childhood, juvenile, early adolescence (preadolescence), true adolescence, adulthood.

- Describe the cognitive development theoretical perspectives of Jean Piaget, Perry, and Belenky *et al.*

- Describe the focus, major concepts, and operating principles of Cognitive Developmental theory:

  Piaget Focused on the processes of thinking and knowing as an invariable sequence of stages that are not necessarily age-linked. Children move through the stages at various paces. Through the processes of assimilation, accommodation, and organization, the child moves through periods of cognitive development. Periods of development with multiple stages:

  - *Sensorimotor Intelligence period* (birth–2 years): Use of reflexes stage; primary circular reactions stage; secondary circular reactions stage; coordination of secondary schemes stage; tertiary circular reactions stage; beginning of thought stage
  - *Preoperational Thought period* (2–7 years): Reorganization, language, beginning logic, egocentrism
  - *Concrete Operations period* (7–11 years): Multiple dimensions, classification, cooperation, tangible, systematic logic
  - *Formal Operations period* (11 years–adulthood): Organize and work systematically in relation to all possibilities

  Perry Focused beyond formal operations as the last stage of cognitive development. Studied young males and identified positions of knowing:

  - *Basic dualism:* Self as passive and authority as knowing, dichotomies
  - *Multiplicity:* One opinion is as good as any other
  - *Relativism subordinate:* Seek out support for opinions
  - *Relativism:* Recognize the truth as relative and varying according to context

  Belenky et al. Focused on the perspectives from which women view the world. Identified five, nonlinear perspectives of knowing:

  - *Silence:* Mindless, voiceless, subject to authority
  - *Received knowledge:* Knowledge comes from authorities, listen to those who know
  - *Subjective knowledge:* Views knowledge as personal, private, intuitive; listens to inner voice; seeks to know self
  - *Procedural knowledge:* Invested in learning and applying information empirically, receives and communicates, seeks the voice of reason, experiences knowledge as both autonomous and in relation to others
  - *Constructed knowledge:* Knowledge is contextual, values both objective and subjective strategies, seeks integration

- Describe the humanistic theoretical perspectives of Abraham Maslow and those of existential philosophers (such as Victor Frankl).

- Describe the focus, major concepts, and operating principles of humanistic and existential theories:

  Maslow Focus on hierarchy of needs to explain motives for human behavior. First two levels are "basic" needs and last three are "growth" needs. Lower-order needs must be met to become self-actualized: Not everyone achieves this goal. Five levels of needs:

  1. Physiological needs
  2. Safety needs
  3. Love and belonging
  4. Esteem and self-esteem
  5. Self-actualization

  Characteristics of the self-actualized person include: tolerance, self-accepting, inner directed, spontaneous, creative, autonomous, caring, capable of intense interpersonal relationships, sense of humor, need for solitude and privacy, and an open attitude toward life.

  Existentialists Many individuals have contributed to the development of existentialism. Basic focus is the view of human beings as continually changing and becoming. Six major existential propositions:

  1. The capacity for self-awareness
  2. Freedom and responsibility
  3. Striving for identity and relationship to others
  4. The search for meaning
  5. Anxiety as a condition of living
  6. Awareness of death and nonbeing.

- Describe the behavioral theoretical perspectives of B. F. Skinner.

- Describe the focus, major concepts, and operating principles of behavioral theory:

  Skinner Focus on overt behavior, how environment affects behavior, and operant conditioning. Behavior occurs because it has been reinforced or is avoided because of negative consequences. Principles of conditioning include:

  - Reinforcement (primary, conditioned)
  - Extinction of behaviors
  - Discriminative stimuli
  - Generalization (of stimulus, of response)
  - Shaping
  - Behavior chains
  - Schedule of reinforcement (random, fixed, continuous, intermittent)
  - Negative reinforcement and punishment
  - Positive reinforcement and reward

- Describe the sociocultural theoretical perspective.

- Describe the focus, major concepts, and operating principles of sociocultural theory. Basic tenet of this school of thought is that any person (or their behavior) can be understood only if consideration is given to the society/culture of their development and that in which they currently live. Eight focal topics of social psychiatry:

1. Social causation
2. Course of mental illness influenced by family, groups, community, and society
3. Treatment and rehabilitation
4. Prevention
5. Governmental and community programs
6. Cultural influences
7. Social control mechanisms
8. Possible existence of a sick society

METHOD

Lecture
Discussion of the application of theories presented in Tables 3-5 through 3-10
Slide/transparency
Reflective thinking exercises

Competency 3.5

Consider various theories as a guide for nursing practice.

CONTENT OUTLINE

- Summarize all theoretical frameworks and content case example/scenario.

METHOD

Discussion of Tables 3-1 through 3-10 (application of theoretical perspectives to case example)
Appendix A

Learning Experiences

Theory Application

- Application of theory about theories is woven throughout the chapter in the case application provided. It is suggested that the educator use these examples in class for discussion and further application of theoretical information.

Individual Activities

- Ask your students to identify one nursing theorist's approach and have them apply it to a client. The students should identify the operating principles and important concepts that are relevant to understanding the client and planning care.

- Direct students to write a paper about the theoretical perspective of one nursing theorist as it applies to current practice of psychiatric mental health nursing.

Group Activities

- Assign three theoretical frameworks randomly among the student cohort of the class. For one day have students respond to all questions from the assigned theoretical perspective. Follow this class with a discussion of how the perspective was facilitating or hindering. Ask students to reflect on how similar/different the perspective was from the framework they tend to use.

Clinical Activities

- In the clinical facility, ask students to identify which theoretical framework provides the basis for the treatment plan that has been developed for an assigned client.

- Over the course of the semester, have the student develop a plan of care for a client using three different theoretical frameworks: developmental, humanistic, and behavioral.

Internet Activities

There are many Internet sites with information about different theoretical perspectives. Below are listed just a few to stimulate discussion.

- Theory and review in psychology can be reached via:

  http://www.gemstate.net/susan/links.htm

- Object relations and psychotherapy can be investigated via:

  http://www.object-relations.com

Neuroscience as Basis for Practice

Chapter 4

Competencies

Upon completion of this chapter, the learner will be able to:

1. Discuss the emerging model of biopsychophysiological theory as an explanation of emotions and behaviors.
2. Explain the major functions of the cerebral lobes, and the diencephalons.
3. Describe modern brain imaging techniques.
4. Explain the role of neurotransmitters, membrane receptors and messenger signaling systems.
5. Discuss the role of genetics in diagnosis and treatment of psychiatric disorders.

Key Terms

Computerized Tomography	Hypothalamus
Cortex	Magnetic Resonance Imaging
Diencephalon	Neurotransmitter
DNA	Positron Emission Tomography
Genetic marker	Thalamus
Genome	

Teaching Methods and Strategies

The medical model which views behavioral and emotional disturbances as an illness is widely accepted within our culture today. Therefore, brain imaging techniques and pharmacological management are mainstays of diagnosis and treatment. It is important for nurses to understand the physiological concepts at the cellular level which undergird this model.

Discoveries in the field of genetics are rapidly changing the way in which the etiology, diagnosis, and treatment of disease (including mental illness) is being approached. Utilizing web sites to explore recent discoveries concerning the genetic versus the environmental risk factors for such conditions as Alzheimer's, schizophrenia, and alcoholism is an excellent way to teach students how to find current information on this topic. Discussions of specific cases in which individuals are making decisions about genetic screening is an excellent way to explore the ethical dilemmas imposed by this new technology. It is also an important way to juxtapose the biopsychophysiological theory with nursing theories as they relate to the way in which behaviors and emotions are viewed in a technological and information-based society.

Lesson Plans

Topic: Neurophysiological basis of behavior and emotion

Competency 4.1

Discuss the emerging model of biopsychological theory as an explanation of emotions and behaviors.

CONTENT OUTLINE

- The neurophysiological theory attributes any symptoms of mental illness to an abnormality in neuroanatomy or neurophysiology. An underlying assumption of this theory is that consciousness, thoughts, emotions, memory, and intuition are the result of neurochemical processes which are under the influence of genetic and environmental factors. Consciousness arises out of the complex neurochemical working of the brain. However, thought and behavior are not solely determined by human biochemistry.

METHOD

Lecture
Slide/transparency

Competency 4.2

Explain the major functions of the cerebral lobes, and the diencephalons.

CONTENT OUTLINE

- Identify components of the diencephalons.
- Discuss the significance of the hypothalamic link between the autonomic nervous system and the endocrine system with regard to behavior and emotion.
- Identify the key areas of the cerebral cortex associated with consciousness and memory as well as the association areas linked with emotions and emotionally mediated behaviors.

METHOD

Lecture
Slide/transparency

Competency 4.3

Describe modern brain imaging techniques.

CONTENT OUTLINE

- CT scans, MRIs, and PET scans permit visualization of the brain.
- CT scans and MRIs are used mainly to diagnose abnormalities of tissue structure such as brain lesions or hematomas.
- PET scans assess brain function and are used to determine whether blood flow, glucose uptake, or binding of neurotransmitters to synaptic membranes is occurring in a normal fashion.

METHOD

Lecture
Slide/transparency

COMPETENCY 4.4

Explain the role of neurotransmitters, membrane receptors and messenger signaling systems.

CONTENT OUTLINE

- Define axon, dendrite, gap junction, and synapse.
- After an action potential has been reached, neurons release neurotransmitters from the end of an axon into the synaptic cleft. The neurotransmitter is taken up by a dendrite where it will cause the opening of ion channels and either stimulate or inhibit nerve function. Most psychiatric medications exert their pharmacological effects directly at the nerve synapse.
- Neurotransmitters bind to a specific receptor and exert their effects directly or through activities of the "second messenger" system.
- Explain how the discovery of various subtypes of cell receptors has improved the treatment of mental illness with pharmacological agents.

METHOD

Lecture
Slide/transparency
Case study

Competency 4.5

Discuss the role of genetics in diagnosis and treatment of psychiatric disorders.

CONTENT OUTLINE

- Advances in chromosome mapping and DNA sequencing hold promise for the identification of the genetic abnormality associated with specific mental illnesses.
- Discuss the way in which mapping techniques and the production of large quantities of DNA may be useful for the diagnosis and treatment of mental illness.

METHOD

Lecture
Slide/transparency

Case study

Learning Experiences

Theory Application

• A case example of genetic screening for Alzheimer's may be given to explore the ethical dilemmas and potential benefits/risks imposed by this type of knowledge and technology.

Individual Activities

• Have the student explain the process by which a neuron transmits the observation of a vehicle rapidly approaching to a muscle; thereby allowing a person the ability to jump out of harm's way.

Have students identify one drug used in the treatment of a specific mental illness that is inhibitory and one that works by stimulating a neural impulse.

Group Activities:

• Debate: Proe and cons of identifying a genetic link to alcholism.

Discuss the question, Should genetic screening be made widely available if such testing is made possible by the discovery of a genetic link to alcoholism? Divide the class into three groups. There will be two debating teams with up to five members and the remainder of the class will be the audience. Faculty will serve as moderator. Flip a coin to choose which team presents first. Each team has 3 minutes to present its comments. Each team then has 5 minutes for rebuttal comments. Finally, each team has 2 minutes for summary statements. After the debate, the audience will discuss the presentation and vote yea or nay.

Clinical Activities

• Review the categories of drugs used to treat depression and explain how the development of drugs which act upon more specific membrane receptor subtypes is usually associated with fewer adverse drug effects.

Community Applications

• Visit the public educational department of a hospital or community health clinic and compare the amount of educational brochures available on the topic of depression as compared with the amount found on the topic of diabetes.

• Interview a high school health or biology teacher to learn how the biophysical basis of mental illness is taught at this level.

Internet Activities

- The Genetics Research Branch of the National Institute of Mental Health can be accessed via:

http://www-grb.nimh.nih.gov

- Read the news release from the American Psychiatric Association on May 1, 2001 which announces the discovery of a genetic link to alcoholism and depression:

http://www.psych.org/news-stand/chromo5101.pdf

NOTES

Diagnostic Systems for Psychiatric Nursing

Chapter 5

Competencies

Upon completion of this chapter, the learner will be able to:

1. Define a diagnostic system and the meaning of a diagnostic taxonomy.
2. Explain the ICD-9 system of medical diagnoses.
3. Explain the DSM diagnostic system, including the meaning of each axis.
4. Explain the use of the NANDA taxonomy in psychiatric mental health nursing practice.
5. Explain the use of the current Nursing Interventions Nursing Outcomes Classification.
6. Describe how information systems affect psychiatric nursing care.

Key Terms

Classification	NANDA	SNOMED
DSM-IV-TR	NIC	UMLS
ICD	NMDS	

Teaching Methods and Strategies

The information about classification systems is often not given emphasis. However, it is important that the nurse fully understand the systems because they are also used for insurance and billing purposes.

The method chosen to present this information varies with the nature of the students' experiences and faculty discretion. Because references with numerical listings are available, the most relevant focus is on the conceptual distinctions and groupings as a whole.

Lesson Plans

Topic: Diagnostic Systems

Competency 5.1

Define a diagnostic system and the meaning of a diagnostic taxonomy.

CONTENT OUTLINE

- Describe the use of classification systems:
  - Categorization
  - Investigate similarities and differences to better understand a phenomenon
  - Systematize language for communications

METHOD

Lecture

Competency 5.2

Explain the ICD-9 system of medical diagnoses.

CONTENT OUTLINE

- Define the International Classification of Disease (ICD) as a comprehensive listing of clinical diagnoses designated by a numerical code.
- Identify how the ICD digital code was changed with the clinical modification for ICD-9-CM.

METHOD

Lecture
Slide/transparency
Case example

Competency 5.3

Explain the DSM diagnostic system, including the meaning of each axis.

CONTENT OUTLINE

- Describe the evolution of the DSM as a system to define criteria needed to confirm diagnosis.
- Describe the DSM-IV multiaxial system approach:
  - *Axis I* Clinical disorder
  - *Axis II* Personality disorders/mental retardation
  - *Axis III* Medical conditions
  - *Axis IV* Psychosocial and environmental problems
  - *Axis V* Global assessment of functioning
- Review the diagnostic categories of the DSM-IV-TR.
- Discuss the pros and cons of the DSM-IV-TR system.
- Compare the DSM-IV-TR and ICD-9-CM systems.

METHOD

Lecture
Discussion
Slide/transparency
Reflective thinking exercises
Case examples

Competency 5.4

Explain the use of the NANDA taxonomy in psychiatric mental health nursing practice.

CONTENT OUTLINE

- Define NANDA nursing diagnoses (a statement of phenomena of concern to nurses that uses human response patterns as an organizing framework).
- Identify the elements of a nursing diagnosis (a diagnostic label, definition, etiology, and defining characteristics).
- Describe the evolution of the NANDA taxonomy of nursing diagnoses.
- Review the human response patterns (display box).
- Relate the NANDA list of nursing diagnoses to the care/concerns of psychiatric nursing practice (display box).
- Discuss the Psychiatric Nursing Diagnoses (PND-1).
- Compare the NANDA, DSM-IV-TR, and ICD-9-CM classification systems.

METHOD

Lecture
Discussion
Slide/transparency
Reflective thinking exercises
Case examples

Competency 5.5

Explain the use of the current Nursing Interventions Nursing Outcomes Classification.

CONTENT OUTLINE

- Describe the purpose of Nursing Interventions Classification (NIC) and Nursing Outcomes Classification (NOC).
- Identify selected nursing interventions that apply to psychiatric nursing (display box).
- Compare the NIC/NOC, NANDA, DSM-IV-TR, and ICD-9-CM classification systems.

METHOD

Lecture
Discussion
Slide/transparency
Reflective thinking exercises
Case example

Competency 5.6

Describe how information systems affect psychiatric nursing care.

CONTENT OUTLINE

- Discuss the trend toward computerization of health records and client care data.
- Clarify the terms related to automated record systems:
  - Information system
  - Computer-based records
  - Computer-based health record
- Discuss the issues of privacy and confidentiality related to automated client records.
- Identify two languaging systems for automated patient records and diagnostic coding:
  - Unified Medical Language System (UMLS)
  - Systematized Nomenclature of Medicine (SNOMED)
- Identify the purpose and requisite components of a Nursing Minimum Data Set (NMDS) (display box).

METHOD

Lecture
Discussion
Slide/transparency
Reflective thinking exercises
Case examples

Learning Experiences

Theory Application

- Building on the examples in the chapter and the reflective thinking exercises, it is suggested that a case example be provided to the class and then go through the process of classification using each system. It is through the application to specific situations that an understanding of the usefulness of the taxonomies evolves.

Individual Activities

- Have students identify the DSM-IV-TR Axis I code for each of the following disorders: Schizophrenia, paranoid type; Dysthymic disorder; Bipolar Disorder with rapid cycling; Panic Disorder without agoraphobia; Attention Deficit Hyperactive Disorder; Post-Traumatic Stress Disorder; Substance abuse, Heroine.

Group Activities

- Debate: Pros and cons of NANDA for nursing care of the mentally ill
- Debate: Pros and cons of DSM-IV-TR for nursing care of the mentally ill

Choose a topic. Divide the class into three groups. There will be two debating teams each with up to five members and the remainder of the class will be the audience. Faculty will serve as moderator. Flip a coin to choose which team presents first. Each team has 3 minutes to present its comments. Each team then has 5 minutes for rebuttal comments. Finally, each team has 2 minutes for summary statements. After the debate, the audience will discuss the presentation and vote yea or nay.

Clinical Activities

- Assign a student to develop a matrix comparing the ICD-9-CM, DSM-IV-TR, and NANDA information related to a specific client.
- Using information about one client, have students discuss information relevant to each classification system.
- Direct students to identify which database/client record system is currently being used in the clinical agency or facility.
- Ask your students to attend clinical rounds and identify which classification system the staff most often uses. For a given client, have students ask for the ICD-9-CM, DSM-IV-TR Axes I–V, and NANDA diagnoses.

Internet Activities

- Access the American Psychiatric Association and information about the DSM-IV-TR:

  http://www.psych.org

- The North American Nursing Diagnosis Association has a web page that discusses the history and purpose of incorporating nursing diagnoses into standardized language systems and health care data bases:

  http://www.NANDA.org

- The University of Iowa, Center for Nursing Classification, has a web site which disseminates current information about the NIC/NOC system:

  http://www.nursing.uiowa.edu/cnc

NOTES

Tools of Psychiatric Mental Health Nursing: Communication, Nursing Process, and the Nurse-Client Relationship

Chapter 6

Competencies

Upon completion of this chapter, the learner will be able to:

1. Describe what is meant by therapeutic use of self.
2. Define verbal and nonverbal communication, giving examples of each.
3. Utilize the skill of therapeutic communication in interactions with clients.
4. Identify various techniques of therapeutic communication, and state when each could be helpful in interactions.
5. Evaluate her own communication with clients.
6. Apply the nursing process in psychiatric settings, emphasizing nursing diagnoses frequently seen in psychiatric care.
7. Identify the phases of the nurse-client relationship.
8. Use the nursing process and a therapeutic nurse-client relationship to provide care.

Key Terms

Defense mechanisms	Process recording
Feedback	Termination phase
Nonverbal communication	Therapeutic communication
Orientation phase	Working phase

Teaching Methods and Strategies

The nursing process, therapeutic communications, and the nurse-client relationship provide the tools for psychiatric mental health nursing practice. Utilizing therapeutic communications in the psychiatric setting requires further skill development, practice, and ongoing, thoughtful analysis of interactions.

Lesson Plans

Topic: Tools of Psychiatric Nursing: Communication, Nursing Process, and Nurse-Client Relationship

Competency 6.1

Describe what is meant by therapeutic use of self.

CONTENT OUTLINE

- Describe the nurse's use of self as an essential feature of the nurse-client relationship.
- Identify the tools of therapeutic self, knowledge of psychiatric theory, and resources in order to offer compassionate care.
- Describe how use of self can facilitate the goals of psychiatric nursing care (control of symptoms, provision of a therapeutic relationship, identification of problems, and interventions to assist the client to attain the best possible state of health).

METHOD

Lecture

Competency 6.2

Define verbal and nonverbal communication, giving examples of each.

CONTENT OUTLINE

- Define therapeutic communication.
- Identify the roles in any interaction (sender and receiver).
- Define effective communication.
- Define feedback and its importance to nursing care.
- Describe types of verbal and nonverbal communications.
- Describe the importance of physical space and room design to the interaction process:

Public space	Personal space
Social space	Intimate space

- Define actions as movements, expressions, gestures, and posture.
- Describe the importance of paralinguistic cues including tone, pitch, volume, sounds, and pace.
- Describe the therapeutic value of touch in communicating.

METHOD

Lecture
Discussion
Slide/transparency
Reflective thinking exercises

Competency 6.3

Utilize the skill of therapeutic communication in interactions with clients.

CONTENT OUTLINE

- Define verbal communication (use of spoken or written words).
- Identify elements needed for communication to be most therapeutic:
  - Conveys respectful attitude
  - Supports individuality of nurse and client
  - Promotes self-esteem for both nurse and client

METHOD

Lecture
Discussion
Slide/transparency
Reflective thinking exercises

Competency 6.4

Identify various techniques of therapeutic communication and state when each could be helpful in interactions.

CONTENT OUTLINE

- Describe the following therapeutic communication techniques:

Listening	Reflection
Silence	Focusing
Broad openings	Informing
Restating	Suggesting
Clarification	Confronting

- Describe, via examples, how and why these techniques may be used (Table 6-1).
- Review the defense mechanisms commonly used in psychiatric settings (Table 6-2).

METHOD

Lecture
Discussion
Slide/transparency
Reflective thinking exercises

Competency 6.5

Evaluate one's own communication with clients.

CONTENT OUTLINE

- Review the importance of evaluation of nurse-client interactions and communications.
- Describe the elements of a process recording.
- Describe how a process recording is useful in facilitating therapeutic communication.

METHOD

Lecture
Slide/transparency

Competency 6.6

Apply the nursing process in psychiatric settings, emphasizing nursing diagnoses frequently seen in psychiatric care.

CONTENT OUTLINE

- Review the nursing process as a problem-solving approach and as a series of actions leading to an end.
- Review the steps of the nursing process and the purpose of each:
  - Assessment
  - Nursing diagnosis
  - Outcome identification
  - Planning/nursing interventions
  - Evaluation
- Identify NANDA nursing diagnoses commonly seen in psychiatric settings (Table 6-5).

METHOD

Lecture
Discussion
Slide/transparency
Reflective thinking exercises

Competency 6.7

Identify the phases of the nurse-client relationship.

CONTENT OUTLINE

- Review the phases of the nurse-client relationship and the nurse's role in each phase:
  - Orientation
  - Working
  - Termination

METHOD

Lecture
Discussion
Slide/transparency
Reflective thinking exercises

Competency 6.8

Use the nursing process and a therapeutic nurse-client relationship to provide care.

CONTENT OUTLINE

- Apply the information about nursing process, nurse-client relationship, and therapeutic communications to a case situation.

METHOD

Discussion

Learning Experiences

Theory Application

- Engage the class in a dialogue about the meaning of the "therapeutic use of self."

• Discuss with the class the behaviors likely to be noted during each phase of the nurse-client relationship.

Individual Activities

• Provide a case example of "an anxious individual" and ask each student to apply the nursing process and formulate a plan of care.

• Provide students with a sample listing of therapeutic techniques and assign them to write one example of each technique.

Group Activities

• Role Play: Using therapeutic communications

Randomly distribute cards to students that identify the primary role as *depressed client* or *psychiatric nurse.* Ask all the "nurses" to gather in a group and discuss and select at least four therapeutic techniques they will use with the client. Simultaneously, request all the "clients" to gather in a group and discuss the behaviors and symptoms they will manifest. Allow approximately 10 minutes for preparation and suggest that students use their notes/textbook for reference. Randomly pair students and have them enact the assigned roles. After 5 minutes of interaction, open the discussion, focusing on communication, the nurse-client relationship, and suggestions. Then have student pairs reverse roles and then evaluate the experience from the other player's perspective.

Clinical Activities

• Have students record an interaction of a staff nurse with a client and analyze the communications using the process recording format.

• Ask your students to observe an intake interview and identify which therapeutic communication techniques facilitate the process for the particular client.

Internet Activities

• Visit:

http://www.gmu.edu/departments/nursing/graduate/duldt/

NOTES

Cultural and Ethnic Considerations

Chapter 7

Competencies

Upon completion of this chapter, the learner will be able to:

1. Define culture as it applies to psychiatric mental health nursing.
2. Discuss the importance of understanding cultural variation when planning and implementing care.
3. Recognize ways in which clients may vary in their beliefs about the health care system and their attitudes about seeking appropriate care.
4. Analyze verbal and nonverbal communication factors that affect transcultural nurse-client interactions.
5. Describe the effect of cultural and ethnic variation on therapeutic management of psychiatric mental health care.

Key Terms

Cultural blindness	Ethnocentrism
Cultural facilitator/broker	Norms
Culture	Stereotyping
Culture shock	Values
Ethnicity	

Teaching Methods and Strategies

Cultural competence requires some level of personal maturity. It is best learned through experiential strategies. However, in order to be able to evaluate one's cultural sensitivity and competence, certain information must be shared. The educator can challenge students to move beyond their own cultural barriers to broaden their view of the world. Then, through discussion and application of information to given situations, understanding of the important nature of cultural and ethnic variables can be facilitated.

It is suggested that the need for cultural sensitivity be incorporated throughout the educational program and linked to every assessment tool that is used. This chapter provides an overview of some of the cultural considerations related to psychiatric mental health nursing practice.

Lesson Plans

Topic: Cultural and Ethnic Considerations

Competency 7.1

Define culture as it applies to psychiatric mental health nursing.

CONTENT OUTLINE

- Define the following terms:
  - Culture
  - Norms
  - Values
  - Ethnocentrism

METHOD

Lecture

Competency 7.2

Discuss the importance of understanding cultural variation when planning and implementing care.

CONTENT OUTLINE

- Describe the elements of cultural competence (Figure 7-1):
  - Cultural awareness
  - Cultural knowledge
  - Cultural skill
  - Cultural encounter
- Describe the elements of ethnicity.
- Identify categories to assess related to cultural variations:
  - Cultural affiliation
  - Values orientation
  - Cultural sanctions and restrictions
  - Communication
  - Health-related beliefs and practices
  - Nutrition
  - Sociocultural considerations
  - Organizations providing cultural support
  - Educational background
  - Religious affiliation
  - Cultural aspects of disease incidence
  - Biocultural variations
  - Developmental considerations
- Discuss the areas to assess related to culturally sensitive mental health care:
  - Beliefs about mental illness and related care
  - Interpersonal interactions
  - Verbal and nonverbal communications
  - Dietary and food habits
  - Biological variation

METHOD

Lecture
Discussion
Slide/transparency
Reflective thinking exercises

Competency 7.3

Recognize ways in which clients may vary in their beliefs about the health care system and their attitudes about seeking appropriate care.

CONTENT OUTLINE

- Discuss the need to determine what behaviors are considered abnormal, for what subgroup, and when.
- Discuss the variations in decisions about when mental health care is sought.
- Discuss the potential cultural barriers to seeking mental health care:
  - Assumptions about mental health
  - Stereotypes of pathology associated with minority lifestyles
  - Ineffective approaches to the values held by minorities
  - Communication/language difficulties

METHOD

Lecture
Discussion
Case example

Competency 7.4

Analyze verbal and nonverbal communication factors that affect transcultural nurse-client interactions.

CONTENT OUTLINE

- Describe some differences in interpersonal interactions that may influence mental health care:
  - Requisite beliefs of inequality of status and power for certain individuals (e.g., rank, gender)
  - Acceptance of collectivism vs. individualism
  - Preference of masculine vs. feminine cultural traits
  - Level of need to avoid uncertainty
  - Meaning of words and behaviors

METHOD

Lecture
Discussion
Case example

Competency 7.5

Describe the effect of cultural and ethnic variation on therapeutic management of psychiatric mental health care.

CONTENT OUTLINE

- Discuss the use of a cultural facilitator to assist in therapeutic management in mental health care.
- Discuss the variations in approach that are related to cultural perspectives about:
  - Verbal communication
  - Nonverbal communication
  - Eye contact
  - Proxemics
  - Touch
  - Silence
  - Social behavior
  - Time orientation

METHOD

Lecture
Discussion
Reflective thinking exercises

Learning Experiences

Theory Application

- Identify three major subgroups of the populace in your area. Provide a list of culturally significant considerations for each subgroup so the students can become familiar with the variables.
- In the classroom setting, ask students to list the perceived variations in verbal and nonverbal communication for individuals with the following ethnic affiliations: Asian, Latino, European, African, Mediterranean, and Native American.

Individual Activities

- Have students identify three personally relevant cultural or ethnic variables and identify how these might facilitate or hinder seeking treatment for a mental disorder such as depression.
- Assign students to discuss with a classmate of differing ethnic or cultural origin how their perceptions about mental illness might vary.

Group Activities

- Seminar: To touch or not to touch, that is the question

  Assign students (five to a group) to investigate the cultural expectations regarding mental health care and the use of touch for specific cultural/ethnic groups common to the locale/region. Each group will select a spokesperson to present their findings to the class. The faculty facilitates discussion by comparing and contrasting the findings of the groups.

Clinical Activities

- Direct students to survey the staff in the clinical agency about the cultural variability of clients and the best approaches to work with these individuals.
- Have the students collaborate with agency staff to develop a list of culture facilitators.

Internet Activities

- Visit the Transcultural Psychiatry home page at McGill University

  http://ww2.mcgill.ca/psychiatry/transcultural/transcult.html
- A need for greater cultural competence in psychiatry was addressed by a symposium sponsored by the American Psychiatric Association:

  http://www.psych.org/pnews/99-12-17/competence.html

- The mission of the National Center for Cultural Competence is to advance the practice of culturally competent care in health care and mental health programs:

  http://gucdc.georgetown.edu/ncc

NOTES

Epidemiology of Mental Health and Illness

Chapter 8

Competencies

Upon completion of this chapter, the learner will be able to:

1. Define epidemiology and describe the major types of epidemiological studies related to mental health.
2. Explain the basic tools of epidemiology, including research tools of descriptive studies, case-controlled studies, and meta-analysis.
3. Discuss the challenges of standardized definitions in mental health.
4. Describe the development of the Diagnostic and Statistical Manual as a means to standardize definitions of psychiatric diagnosis.
5. Cite data from early epidemiological studies, the Epidemiological Catchment Area Study, and the National Comorbidity Study (NCS) to demonstrate understanding of the incidence and prevalence of mental illness in the United States.

Key Terms

Blinded clinical trial	Interrater agreement
Case-control study	Interrater reliability
Cohort study	Intrarater reliability
Control group	Longitudinal study
Controlled clinical trials	Meta-analysis
Descriptive study	Placebo
Double-blinded trial	Prevalence
Endemic	Quasi-experimental study
Epidemic	Reliability
Epidemiology	Risk factors
Experimental group	Validity
Incidence	

Teaching Methods and Strategies

The content in Chapter 8 presents a challenge to the educator. Some may find it inherently interesting while others find it dry and unappealing. However, for the student to function in a manner that demonstrates critical thinking, the information provides a framework for understanding psychiatric nursing care.

If a separate course is included in the curriculum that emphasizes design and research elements, then the educator may elect to spend far less time covering this content. The student could be held accountable for reviewing Chapter 8 content in an independent manner.

Lesson Plans

Topic: Epidemiology

Competency 8.1

Define epidemiology.

CONTENT OUTLINE

- Define the terms *epidemiology, epidemic, endemic, incidence, prevalence, validity,* and *reliability.*
- Describe the focus/purpose of conducting epidemiological studies.

METHOD

Lecture
Slide/transparency

Competency 8.2

Explain the basic tools of epidemiology, including research tools of descriptive studies, case-controlled studies, and meta-analysis.

CONTENT OUTLINE

- Describe meta-analysis.
- Describe the following types of studies:

Descriptive	Longitudinal
Quasi-experimental	Cohort
Case-controlled	Controlled clinical

METHOD

Lecture
Slide/transparency

Competency 8.3

Discuss the challenges of standardized definitions in mental health.

CONTENT OUTLINE

- Discuss the issue of rating the degrees of mental illness or symptoms.
- Define the terms *interrater reliability* and *intrarater reliability.*

METHOD

Lecture
Slide/transparency

Competency 8.4

Describe the development of the Diagnostic and Statistical Manual as a means to standardize definitions of psychiatric diagnosis.

CONTENT OUTLINE

- Describe the process used in developing the diagnostic criteria in the DSM.
- Describe how interrater reliability and intrarater reliability were used in the development of the DSM criteria for diagnosis of mental disorders.

METHOD

Lecture

Competency 8.5

Cite data from early epidemiological studies and the Epidemiological Catchment Area (ECA) Study to demonstrate understanding of the incidence and prevalence of mental illness in the United States.

CONTENT OUTLINE

- Identify the most important outcome of early epidemiological studies of mental illness.
- Discuss the purpose of the Epidemiological Catchment Area (ECA) Study.
- Describe the steps in carrying out the ECA Study.
- Discuss the findings of the National Comorbidity Study (NCS).
- Describe the "tip-of-the-iceberg" phenomenon and its importance to psychiatric mental health nursing.

METHOD

Lecture
Discussion
Reflective thinking exercises

Learning Experiences

Theory Application

• To demonstrate the concepts of epidemiology as well as the tip-of-the-iceberg phenomenon, engage the class in a four-part exercise.

Part I: Have the class develop five questions about the prevalence of personal experiences with mental illness.

Part II: Each student will complete the survey anonymously. A student volunteer will collect this information and the responses will be summarized. Only grouped data will be shared.

Part III: Each student is to collect the same survey information from any two other people (not enrolled in a nursing class) and bring it to the next class session where data will be summarized and grouped data shared.

Part IV: The summary results from parts II and III will be compared. Then data will be combined and the combined results will be compared with the two separate survey summaries. Discuss the outcomes in light of the concepts of epidemiology.

Individual Activities

• Assign students to review two psychiatric nursing journals and identify the number of articles that relate to the epidemiology of mental illness.

• Direct students to use the DSM-IV-TR to find information about the incidence of the following disorders: Mood disorders, Schizophrenia, Anxiety disorders, and Substance-use disorders.

Group Activities

• To demonstrate the difficulties in developing criteria for evaluating mental illness or health, divide the students into two groups. Each group is to discuss and decide on three to five criteria that indicate that a person is mentally healthy. A spokesperson from each group will share the criteria. Discuss the process and the similarities or differences in the selected criteria.

• Discussion: How would you study the question "Can mental illness be prevented?"

Apply the epidemiological concepts presented in this chapter.

Clinical Activities

• Ask students to evaluate the impact of mental illness for clients in the clinical setting using the question "How much difficulty does mental illness cause?" (from the Carter Commission on Mental Health). Note the variability in responses and the qualifying information associated with each person's response.

• Focusing on the current client diagnostic mix in the clinical facility where the students are assigned, have them identify the epidemiological information about three psychiatric diagnoses.

Internet Activities

• The Department of Epidemiology and Service Research of the National Institute of Mental Health can be accessed via:

http://www.nimh.nih.gov/dsir/ index.cfm

• The home page for the National Mental Health Association discusses the work of this organization which is to improve the mental health of all Americans through advocacy, education, research, and service:

http://nmha.wego.com

Ethical and Legal Bases for Care

Chapter 9

Competencies

Upon completion of this chapter, the learner will be able to:

1. Describe the legal parameters and nursing responsibilities related to clients' rights; confidentiality; psychological competence; informed consent; right to refuse treatment; involuntary hospitalization; professional negligence; violent or self-destructive clients.
2. Define the ethical theories of utilitarianism and deontology.
3. Identify the principles that guide practice decisions in psychiatric mental health nursing, including autonomy, beneficence, fidelity, justice, and nonmaleficence.
4. Use the Value Analysis model for evaluation of ethical dilemmas.

Key Terms

Abandonment	Least restrictive alternative
Autonomy	Malpractice
Beneficence	M'Naghten test
Civil commitment	Negligence
Code of ethics	Nonmaleficence
Competency to stand trial	Normative ethics
Conservator	Physical restraint
Deontology	Probate proceedings
Emergency hospitalization	Seclusion
Ethics	Tarasoff duty to warn
Fidelity	Utilitarianism
Incompetence	
Justice	

Teaching Methods and Strategies

The importance of practice guided by a code of ethics is the focus of this chapter. Assisting the student to understand the ethical parameters of professional practice and the legal boundaries of care is a challenge. Within the chapter are reflective exercises and questions to stimulate consideration of the ethics of psychiatric mental health nursing practice.

Lesson Plans

Topic: Ethical and Legal Bases for Care

Competency 9.1

Describe the legal parameters and nursing responsibilities related to clients' rights; confidentiality; psychological competence; informed consent; right to refuse treatment; involuntary hospitalization; professional negligence; violent or self-destructive clients.

CONTENT OUTLINE

- Define ethics as the philosophical considerations and principles guiding human interactions.
- Define the following terms:
  - Confidentiality
  - Privacy
  - Psychological competence
  - Involuntary hospitalization
  - Informed consent
  - Right to refuse treatment
  - Least restrictive care
- Discuss the legal elements related to the aforementioned terms, including the M'Naghten test and the Tarasoff duty to warn.
- Describe situations that might indicate professional negligence:
  - Failure to warn
  - Failure to recognize suicidal risk
  - Sexual involvement
  - Breaching confidentiality
  - Failure to honor individual rights
  - Failure to use the least restrictive alternative
  - Failure to protect
- Discuss the ethical dilemmas that arise due to patients' rights and professional responsibilities.

METHOD

Lecture
Discussion
Slide/transparency
Reflective thinking exercises

Competency 9.2

Define the ethical theories of utilitarianism and deontology.

CONTENT OUTLINE

- Define utilitarianism (the greatest good for the greatest number).
- Define deontology (human duty to others).

- Describe the deontological principles of autonomy, beneficence, fidelity, justice, and nonmaleficence.
- Compare these two ethical perspectives.

METHOD

Lecture
Discussion
Slide/transparency
Reflective thinking exercises

Competency 9.3

Identify the principles that guide practice decisions in psychiatric mental health nursing, including autonomy, beneficence, fidelity, justice, and nonmaleficence.

CONTENT OUTLINE

- Define autonomy, beneficence, fidelity, justice, and nonmaleficence.
- Discuss how these principles guide care decisions and nursing practice.
- Discuss why the principle of justice is less prominent than other principles in the psychiatric mental health arena.

METHOD

Lecture
Discussion
Slide/transparency

Competency 9.4

Use the Value Analysis model for evaluation of ethical dilemmas.

CONTENT OUTLINE

- Describe the focus of the Value Analysis model for evaluating ethical dilemmas.
- Identify the steps in the Value Analysis model.
- Apply the Value Analysis model to a case example.

METHOD

Lecture
Discussion
Case example

Learning Experiences

Theory Application

- Have students use the ethical theories of utilitarianism and deontology to compare and contrast the legal and ethical issues central to psychiatric mental health nursing (suggestion is to use a matrix format).

Individual Activities

- Direct students to reflect on which of the principles of deontology is the most important to them as an individual and have them briefly describe why in a journal.
- Throughout the psychiatric nursing experience, ask students to record (in a journal) their perspective on the ethical dilemmas encountered. At the end of the experience, have the students reflect on these and consider if their perspectives have in any way changed.

Group Activities

- Discussion: The right to refuse treatment

  Use the reflective thinking case example of Mrs. Wenzel (right to refuse treatment). Instruct students to discuss the situation using each of the Supreme Court's considerations for treatment against one's will.
- Divide the students into three groups to investigate the following: (1) the state's nurse practice act information about negligence; (2) the state codes regarding involuntary hospitalization; (3) state's guidelines for psychological competency. Have each group write a short report of the findings to be shared with the class.

Clinical Activities

- In the clinical area, identify at least two ethical dilemmas and have students discuss them from the perspective of deontology and utilitarianism.
- Identify the agency/facility procedures for utilizing seclusion and restraints. Are there specific guidelines for making these decisions?

Internet Activities

Several courses and educational offerings dealing with ethics and the legal aspects of mental illness can be found on the Internet. In addition, there are numerous listings of books, periodicals, and abstracts dealing with these topics.

- Code of ethics published by the American Nurses Association (ANA)

  http://nursingworld.org/ajn/2000/july/issues.htm
- A Mental Health Patient's Bill of Rights published by the American Psychological Association which focuses on managed care and insurance issues:

  http://www.apa.org/spreadtheword/rights.html

Unit 2

Clients with Psychiatric Disorders

The ten chapters in Unit 2 provide substantial information about the major mental illnesses. The disorders described by the DSM-IV-TR largely fall within the content of these chapters.

A major thrust of each chapter is the application of the nursing process to caring for the client with the disorder or groups of disorders that are the focus of the particular chapter. The case examples, care plans, and personal descriptions of the lived experiences related to the disorder provide excellent teaching tools. The learning activities at the end of each section also include suggestions for community applications related to the specific clinical diagnoses.

NOTES

The Client Undergoing Crisis

Chapter 10

Competencies

Upon completion of this chapter, the learner will be able to:

1. Identify crisis as part of life and describe situations that bring on crisis for many individuals.
2. Describe situational, maturational, cultural, and community crises.
3. Identify four phases of a person's experience with crisis.
4. Use stress theory to interpret an individual's response to crisis.
5. Identify daily stressors in modern life that produce personal stress and require adaptive responses.
6. Use the adaptation nursing theories of Roy and Erickson's Modeling and Role-Modeling theory to evaluate the crisis response, adaptation, and return to an equilibrium state.
7. Use the caring, interpersonal nursing theories of Watson and Peplau to seek to understand the client's subjective experience of the crisis event and provide unconditional, humanistic care.
8. Use Cultural Care theory to obtain knowledge of the client's culture and to understand the meaning of life's events from within that culture.
9. Apply the nursing process to the care of clients in crisis.

Key Terms

Adaptive energy
Adaptive potential assessment model
Arousal
Community crisis
Conservative-withdrawal state
Crisis
Cultural crisis
Culture shock
Equilibrium
Fight-flight response
General Adaptation Syndrome
Impoverishment
Maturational crisis
Psychological development
Situational crisis
Stress

Teaching Methods and Strategies

As with many of the topics encountered during the study of psychiatric nursing, crisis is most fully understood from the lived experience. The perspective set forth in Chapter 10 evolves from a stress and adaptation model. In this sense, all humans experience some degree of crisis. For educational purposes, the types of crises, the stages of crisis, and application of several nursing theories have been included.

Lesson Plans

Topic: Crisis

Competency 10.1

Identify crisis as a part of life and describe situations that bring on crisis for many individuals.

CONTENT OUTLINE

- Define crisis.

METHOD

Lecture

Competency 10.2

Describe situational, maturational, cultural, and community crises.

CONTENT OUTLINE

- Define the terms:
  - Situational crisis
  - Maturational crisis
  - Cultural crisis
  - Community crisis
- Identify at least two examples of each type of crisis.

METHOD

Lecture
Slide/transparency

Competency 10.3

Identify four phases of a person's experience of crisis.

CONTENT OUTLINE

- Describe the first phase of crisis: threat.
- Describe the second phase of crisis: increased anxiety with decreased coping ability.
- Describe the third phase of crisis: escalating anxiety.
- Describe the fourth phase of anxiety: panic.

METHOD

Lecture
Slide/transparency
Case example

Competency 10.4

Use stress theory to interpret an individual's response to crisis.

CONTENT OUTLINE

- Define stress.
- Describe the General Adaptation Syndrome (Selye) as a response to stress.
- Describe the fight-flight response to stress.

METHOD

Lecture

Competency 10.5

Identify daily stressors in modern life that produce personal stress and require adaptive responses.

CONTENT OUTLINE

- Review the list of modern day stressors that are often experienced.

METHOD

Lecture

Competency 10.6

Use the adaptation nursing theories of Roy and Erickson's Modeling and Role-Modeling theory to evaluate the crisis response, adaptation, and return to an equilibrium state.

CONTENT OUTLINE

- Discuss the components of the nursing adaptation theories: Roy—biological, psychological, and sociological; Erickson—biophysical, cognitive, psychological, sociological.
- Describe the Adaptation Potential Assessment model and the associated phenomena (Figures 10-1 and 10-2).
- Identify the nursing actions for dealing with crises that arise from the adaptation theories: establish trust; identify strengths; promote positive orientation and perceived control.

METHOD

Lecture
Slide/transparency

Competency 10.7

Use the caring, interpersonal nursing theories of Watson and Peplau to seek to understand the client's subjective experience of the crisis event and provide unconditional, humanistic care.

CONTENT OUTLINE

- Describe the focus of caring nursing theories as applied to crisis situations.
- Identify relevant nursing actions from a caring theoretical framework: listening, sincerity, unconditional acceptance, understanding subjective experience, assisting client to interpret themes and meaning of the crisis.

METHOD

Lecture
Slide/transparency

Competency 10.8

Use Cultural Care theory to obtain knowledge of the client's culture and to understand the meaning of life's events from within that culture.

CONTENT OUTLINE

- Describe the focus of Cultural Care theory in dealing with a crisis situation.
- Identify the best method to assess the individual's culture and meaning of the crisis.

METHOD

Lecture
Slide/transparency

Competency 10.9

Apply the nursing process to the care of clients in crisis.

CONTENT OUTLINE

- Review the assessment questions for a client in crisis.
- Review Figure 10-5, The Adaptive Potential, as a guide for nursing interventions.
- Identify nursing diagnoses common to clients in crisis: anxiety, fear, ineffective coping, powerlessness, hopelessness, etc.
- Link the outcome identification and planned interventions to the selected nursing diagnoses.
- Review/discuss the case study care plan provided in the chapter.

METHOD

Lecture
Discussion
Slide/transparency
Case example

Learning Experiences

Theory Application

- Using the following case example, have students apply the theories related to crisis and the nursing process to develop a plan of care. The client is a 23-year-old woman who survived a car accident that killed her father and twin sibling. She is in the hospital, in stable condition, and has begun to show obvious signs of psychological crisis associated with her case.

Individual Activities

- Ask students to identify a time when they, or a close family member, experienced a crisis. How did they respond?

• In their journals, have students indicate the feelings they experienced when reading "Everything in its Path," and consider how this would influence how they would provide nursing care in this situation.

Group Activities

• Discussion: APAM

Instruct the group to apply the Adaptation Potential Assessment model to a scenario as a group. Discuss the phenomena to assess for each state.

Scenario: J. D.'s girlfriend has told him she doesn't want to see him anymore. He doesn't want to live without her. He's missed the last three days at work. He comes to the emergency room complaining of nausea, shortness of breath, profuse sweating, and heart palpitations

• Discussion: How to best respond

Using a group brainstorming and problem-solving approach, analyze the preceding scenario to identify (1) the central or immediate problem; (2) contributing factors; (3) main nursing diagnosis; (4) outcomes; and (5) nursing interventions.

Clinical Activities

• Identify the crisis support resources available to clients.

• Encourage students to interview a nurse who works at a crisis center.

• Trends and shifts in health care may mean changes in the role of the nurse. What crisis situations might you anticipate for the nursing profession?

Community Applications

• Look up the crisis listings in the local community telephone directory and develop a reference card to share at a community health fair.

• In cooperation with a local high school, arrange to have a booth for teen crisis information at a health fair.

Internet Activities

• Crisis intervention resources web site:

http://www.crisis.org

NOTES

The Client Experiencing Anxiety

Chapter 11

Competencies

Upon completion of this chapter, the learner will be able to:

1. Understand the objective experience of the emotion of anxiety.
2. Describe the differences between anxiety and fear.
3. Define and describe six major anxiety disorders (Generalized Anxiety Disorder, Panic Disorder, Agoraphobia, Phobias, Obsessive-Compulsive Disorder, and Post-Traumatic Stress Disorder).
4. Relate the prevalence of anxiety disorders in the general population.
5. Participate in the major treatments of clients with anxiety disorders, including psychotherapy, medication, and combination treatment.
6. Apply nursing theory and nursing diagnoses in the planning, implementing, and evaluating of nursing care of clients with anxiety disorders.

Key Terms

Adversity	Fear	Positron emission tomography (PET)
Agoraphobia	Generalized Anxiety Disorder	Post-Traumatic Stress Disorder
Anxiety	Obsession	Trait anxiety
Cognitive-behavior therapy	Panic Disorder	
Compulsion	Phobia	

Teaching Methods and Strategies

As with all the chapters in Unit 2, the methods and strategies used to teach the information relies heavily on utilizing the nursing process. The case examples and case care plans in this chapter lend themselves to a variety of applications. In addition, it is suggested that the DSM-IV-TR itself be incorporated as a teaching strategy to add specificity to the content of the chapter.

Lesson Plans

Topic: Anxiety

Competency 11.1

Understand the objective experience of the emotion of anxiety.

CONTENT OUTLINE

- Describe the manifestations of anxiety.
- Describe the neurobiology of anxiety.

METHOD

Lecture

Competency 11.2

Describe the differences between anxiety and fear.

CONTENT OUTLINE

- Define fear.
- Define anxiety.
- Describe the stages of anxiety (Table 11-1).

METHOD

Lecture
Slide/transparency

Competency 11.3

Define and describe six major anxiety disorders:

1. Generalized Anxiety Disorder
2. Panic Disorder
3. Agoraphobia
4. Phobias
5. Obsessive-Compulsive Disorder
6. Post-Traumatic Stress Disorder.

CONTENT OUTLINE

- Define and describe the symptoms of Generalized Anxiety Disorder:
  - Restlessness
  - Fatigue
  - Difficulty concentrating
  - Irritability
  - Muscle tension
  - Sleep disturbances
- Define and describe the symptoms associated with Panic Disorder:
  - Palpitations
  - Sweating
  - Tremors
  - Shortness of breath
  - Chest pain
  - Fear of losing control
  - Fear of dying
  - Altered sense of reality
- Define and describe the symptoms of Agoraphobia:
  - Intense feelings of anxiety that result in refraining from going out and avoiding situations
- Define and describe the symptoms of Phobia:
  - Persistent fear of a specific object or situation that interferes with life activities
- Define and describe the symptoms of Obsessive-Compulsive Disorder:
  - Obsessional thoughts
  - Compulsion to act
  - Recognizes the thoughts and actions are unreasonable but cannot refrain

- Define and describe the symptoms associated with Post-Traumatic Stress Disorder:

Recurrent recollections	Nightmares
Flashbacks	Impaired functioning

METHOD

Lecture
Slide/transparency
Review Table 11-2

Competency 11.4

Relate the prevalence of anxiety disorders in the general population.

CONTENT OUTLINE

- Identify the prevalence (percentage of the adult population of the United States that experience) of anxiety disorders.
- Compare the different prevalence rates for the aforementioned anxiety-related disorders.

METHOD

Lecture
Slide/transparency

Competency 11.5

Participate in the major treatments of clients with anxiety disorders, including psychotherapy, medication, and combination treatment.

CONTENT OUTLINE

- Describe the use of psychotherapy to treat anxiety disorders.
- Describe the use of cognitive-behavioral therapy to treat anxiety disorders and victims of traumatic events.
- Describe the use of pharmacotherapy to treat anxiety disorders.
- Describe the use of combination therapy in the treatment of anxiety disorders.

METHOD

Lecture
Slide/transparency

Competency 11.6

Apply nursing theory and nursing diagnoses in the planning, implementing, and evaluating of nursing care of clients with anxiety disorders.

CONTENT OUTLINE

- Discuss the importance of trust in the care of the client with anxiety disorder.
- Discuss screening for anxiety disorders.
- Identify nursing diagnoses associated with anxiety disorders:

Anxiety	Ineffective coping
Fear	Sleep pattern disturbance
Interrupted family processes	

- Review the case study care plan for this chapter.

METHOD

Lecture
Discussion
Case example

Learning Experiences

Theory Application

- Use the DSM-IV-TR decision tree for anxiety-related disorders to compare the different disorders noted in this chapter.
- Using an educational video, review the different behaviors and treatments for anxiety-related disorders.

Individual Activities

- Ask students to review a standard plan of care for Agoraphobia.
- Have students list all the possible nursing diagnoses that apply to the diagnosis of Phobia, specific (client fears electricity).

Group Activities

- Discussion: Should the nursing care for the person diagnosed with agoraphobia with panic disorder be different from the care for a person diagnosed with agoraphobia without panic disorder?
- Discussion: How do the actions of the nonbenzodiazepine drugs differ from the benzodiazepines used for the treatment of anxiety disorders?

Clinical Activities

- Review the procedures for systematic desensitization used in treatment of phobias.
- In the clinical area, review the behaviors of a client diagnosed with an anxiety disorder and compare them to the DSM-IV-TR criteria for diagnoses.

Community Applications

- Contact the community health department or designated county health department and request a list of resources available for the person diagnosed with an anxiety disorder.
- Visit the local library and identify at least two references available to the public regarding anxiety disorders.

Internet Activities

- Information, news, treatment approaches, and other links related to anxiety and anxiety disorders can be found on tAPir, the Anxiety Panic Internet resource:

  http://www.algy.com/anxiety

- General information about anxiety disorders and related issues can be located at the Anxiety-Panic Resources page provided by the Panic Disorder Institute:

  http://www.anxiety-panic.com

The Client Experiencing Schizophrenia

Chapter 12

Competencies

Upon completion of this chapter, the learner will be able to:

1. Compare altered thought processes as normal human responses to the psychiatric conditions schizophrenia and psychosis.
2. Empathize with the lived experiences of those who have schizophrenia and those who have a family member with the condition.
3. Recognize the presenting symptoms of schizophrenia.
4. Discuss the epidemiology of schizophrenia.
5. Explain the etiology of schizophrenia as an organic disease.
6. Discuss the genetic factors known with regard to the transition of schizophrenia.
7. Engage in psychosocial therapeutic treatments for individuals and their families.
8. Explain the role of neuroleptic drugs in the management of schizophrenia.
9. Provide nursing care to persons suffering from schizophrenia, based on nursing theory and nursing process.

Key Terms

Akathisia
Akinesia
Alogia
Anhedonia
Avolition
Catatonia
Delusion
Derailment
Dystonia
Flattened affect
Grandiose delusion
Hallucination
Incoherence
Neologistic word
Persecutory delusion
Psychotic
Referential delusion
Schizophrenia
Tangentiality
Tardive dyskinesia
Word salad

Teaching Methods and Strategies

Understanding the complexities of the schizophrenic's experiences is no easy task. Experience in dealing with a schizophrenic client provides the best learning opportunities. There are many video and media productions available to enhance the teaching of this content.

The case examples and the care plan featured in this chapter provide excellent resources to the educator. In addition, it is suggested that the DSM-IV-TR itself be used to provide more depth to the information about the clinical features and symptoms associated with schizophrenia.

Lesson Plans

Topic: Schizophrenia

Competency 12.1

Compare altered thought processes as normal human responses to the psychiatric conditions of schizophrenia and psychosis.

CONTENT OUTLINE

- Describe schizophrenia and psychosis.
- Describe two myths about schizophrenia.

METHOD

Lecture

Competency 12.2

Empathize with the lived experiences of those who have schizophrenia and those who have a family member with the condition.

CONTENT OUTLINE

- Discuss perceptions of the experiences of a person diagnosed as schizophrenic and his/her family members' experiences.

METHOD

Discussion
Case example
Review: "Anonymous Autobiography"

Competency 12.3

Recognize the presenting symptoms of schizophrenia.

CONTENT OUTLINE

- Describe the features associated with schizophrenia and psychoses:
  - Disordered thoughts (loose association, flight of ideas)
  - Language disturbances (neologism, word salad, tangentiality, incoherence)

Loss of function (diminished personal hygiene, not able to maintain social norms, catatonia)
Delusions (grandiose, persecutory, referential)
Hallucinations (auditory, visual, tactile, olfactory)

- Describe the "negative" symptoms associated with schizophrenia and psychoses:

Flattened affect	Avolition
Alogia	Anhedonia

- Describe the clinical course of schizophrenia.

METHOD

Lecture
Slide/transparency
Case example

Competency 12.4

Discuss the epidemiology of schizophrenia.

CONTENT OUTLINE

- Identify the major challenge for epidemiologists regarding schizophrenia.
- Describe the social and financial impact of schizophrenia.

METHOD

Lecture
Slide/transparency

Competency 12.5

Explain the etiology of schizophrenia as an organic disease.

CONTENT OUTLINE

- Describe the recent findings of anatomical and physiologic differences in the brains of schizophrenics.
- Describe the role of imaging techniques in the search for organic causes of schizophrenia.
- Describe the dopamine hypothesis of schizophrenia.
- Emphasize that the definitive etiology of schizophrenia is still *unknown*.

METHOD

Lecture
Slide/transparency

Competency 12.6

Discuss the genetic factors known with regard to the transition of schizophrenia.

CONTENT OUTLINE

- Describe the supporting results of twin studies.
- Identify the inheritance of predisposition for developing schizophrenia.

METHOD

Lecture

Competency 12.7

Engage in psychosocial therapeutic treatments for individuals and their families.

CONTENT OUTLINE

- Identify psychotherapeutic treatments for schizophrenia.
- Describe psychosocial and family support services for clients diagnosed with schizophrenia.
- Describe the rehabilitation efforts for persons with schizophrenia.

METHOD

Lecture
Slide/transparency

Competency 12.8

Explain the role of neuroleptic drugs in the management of schizophrenia.

CONTENT OUTLINE

- Discuss the role of psychopharmacology in the management of symptoms of schizophrenia.
- Describe the major mechanism of action of the antipsychotic medications.
- Describe the major side effects and adverse responses of antipsychotic medications:
  Acute dystonia
  Akathisia
  Akinesia
  Tardive dyskinesia
  Neuroleptic Malignant Syndrome
  Anticholinergic effects

METHOD

Lecture
Slide/transparency
Handout

Competency 12.9

Provide nursing care to persons suffering from schizophrenia, based on nursing theory and nursing process.

CONTENT OUTLINE

- Identify the major nursing diagnoses associated with schizophrenia:
  Disturbed thought processes
  Disturbed sensory perceptions
  Impaired verbal communication
  Ineffective role performance
  Self-care deficit
  Social isolation
- Describe the basic nursing interventions that promote trust, positive orientation, perceived control, strengths, and meet health-directed goals.

• Review the assessment parameters for schizophrenic clients.

METHOD

Lecture
Discussion
Slide/transparency
Case example

Learning Experiences

Theory Application

• Use the DSM-IV-TR decision tree for psychotic disorders to compare the different disorders.

• Using an educational video, review the different behaviors and treatments for schizophrenia.

Individual Activities

• Have students review a standard plan of care for Schizophrenia, paranoid type.

• Encourage students to review all the types of schizophrenia described in the DSM-IV-TR.

Group Activities

• Discussion: How functional are most schizophrenics and what role does medication and compliance play in this?

• Discussion: How do the actions of the new antipsychotic drugs differ from the traditional neuroleptic medications?

Clinical Activities

• Review the procedures for ECT, sometimes used in treatment of schizophrenia.

• In the clinical area, review the behaviors of a client diagnosed with schizophrenia and compare them to the DSM-IV-TR criteria for the diagnosis.

Community Applications

• Identify one community psychosocial program and identify the mission statement.

• Contact the community health department or designated county health department and request a list of resources available for schizophrenic patients and their significant others/family members.

Internet Activities

• Visit the Schizophrenia home page for information about this disorder, neuropathology, management, and more:

http://www.schizophrenia.com

• The IMH Network has links for schizophrenia, biological research, and media:

http://www.ptan.com/links/link23.htm

• Visit the National Alliance for Research on Schizophrenia and Depression website:

http://www.mhsource.com/narsad

NOTES

The Client Experiencing Depression

Chapter 13

Competencies

Upon completion of this chapter, the learner will be able to:

1. Identify mood swings as a normal part of the human emotional experience.
2. Employ empathy to understand one's own experience of depression and to understand the depressive feelings of others.
3. Define depression and differentiate between major and minor depressive disorders.
4. Describe the concepts of grief and bereavement.
5. Analyze predisposing factors to grief and depression.
6. Identify major psychological theories that explain depression.
7. Integrate a nursing theory base into care for depressed clients.
8. Apply the nursing process to the care of clients who are depressed.

Key Terms

Bipolar depression	Marital therapy
Brief dynamic therapy	Masked grief
Chronic grief	Mood disorder
Cognitive therapy	Mood episode
Delayed grief	Nurse agency
Depression	Self-care agency
Ego	Superego
Exaggerated grief	Supportive-educative role
Grief	Unipolar depression

Teaching Methods and Strategies

There are numerous methods that may be used to expand the students' understanding of depression and how to provide quality nursing care to the depressed client. Because the problems of depression are reported in at least 10% of the population, most students will have had some experience with someone who has demonstrated depressive symptoms. It is useful to engage the students in providing examples and to use the examples to highlight the associated symptoms and therapeutic approaches. If time permits, discussion and group problem solving might be used. If time is limited, providing synthesis of the content will help the students understand the content.

Lesson Plans

Topic: Depression

Competency 13.1

Identify mood swings as a normal part of the human emotional experience.

CONTENT OUTLINE

- Discuss the notion that mood swings are a part of everyone's life.
- Discuss that emotion means to experience a range of feelings.

METHOD

Lecture

Competency 13.2

Employ empathy to understand one's own experience of depression and to understand the depressive feelings of others.

CONTENT OUTLINE

- Discuss empathy and the experience of empathy in nursing care of the depressed person.

METHOD

Discussion focused on literature excerpts in this chapter: *Written on Seeing the Flowers*; *Amalia*; *My Confessions*; *The Crack-Up*.

Competency 13.3

Define depression and differentiate between major and minor depressive disorders.

CONTENT OUTLINE

- Review the DSM-IV-TR criteria for Major Depressive Disorder.
- Review the criteria for Minor Depression.
- Review the DSM-IV-TR criteria for Dysthymic Disorder.

METHOD

Lecture

Competency 13.4

Describe the concepts of grief and bereavement.

CONTENT OUTLINE

- Discuss the dynamics of grief and bereavement as normal:
  - Feelings of loss and sadness
  - May take up to 3 years to resolve and exhibit adaptive behaviors
- Describe the stages of the normal grieving process:
  - Stage I: Period of shock
  - Stage II: Reality stage
  - Stage III: Recovery stage
- Describe the experience of abnormal grieving:
  - Chronic grief
  - Exaggerated grief
  - Delayed grief
  - Masked grief

METHOD

Lecture
Slide/transparency

Competency 13.5

Analyze predisposing factors to grief and depression.

CONTENT OUTLINE

- Delineate the risk factors for depression:
  - Family history
  - Recent negative stressors
  - Childhood in negative home environment
  - Lack of social support system
  - Having significant physical disorder
- Describe factors that lead to abnormal grief:
  - Ambivalence toward the person lost
  - Unresolved emotional conflicts with relationship
  - History of maladaptive coping behaviors

METHOD

Lecture
Slide/transparency

Competency 13.6

Identify major psychological theories that explain depression.

CONTENT OUTLINE

- Describe the Freudian basis for psychoanalytical theoretical perspectives of depression:
  - Conflict between ego and superego
  - Resultant guilt, self-hate, anger turned inward
- Describe other theories of depression:
  - *Object loss theory* (Bowlby): Emerged from psychoanalysis, depression is due to traumatic loss early in life and subsequent loss/separation in adulthood.
  - *Learned helplessness theory* (Seligman): Sense that one has no control over life events and develops a personality of "giving up."
  - *Cognitive theory* (Beck): In opposition to analytical perspective, focusing on how person thinks:
    - – Accepting faulty thought processes to hold to dysfunctional beliefs
    - – Irrational beliefs about self and world causes painful emotions and maladaptive behaviors
- Describe the psychobiological premise of depression—depression is at some level a disease of the brain.
  - Monoamine concentrations in the brain (especially serotonin & norepinephrine) play a role in depressive symptoms
  - Consistent changes in metabolic functioning of the frontal and temporal lobes
  - Increased amygdala activity
- Identify treatment approaches to deal with depression:
  - Psychotherapies
    - – Brief therapy
    - – Marital therapy
    - – Cognitive therapy
  - Physical (somatic) therapies
    - – Electroconvulsive therapy
    - – Phototherapy
    - – Medications (antidepressants)
      - Tricyclics
      - Selective serotonin reuptake inhibitors
      - Selective norepinephrine reuptake inhibitors
      - Monoamine oxidase inhibitors
      - St. John's Wort

METHOD

Lecture
Slide/transparency
Review Table 13-1 and "Foods and Medications that must be Avoided by Clients taking MAO Inhibitors"

Competency 13.7

Integrate a nursing theory base into care for depressed clients.

CONTENT OUTLINE

- Describe the perspective of Caring theory for care of the depressed person:
  - Focus of changing isolation and loneliness symptoms
  - Value the individual, seek to understand the experience, provide respect, nurturing, and support
- Describe the perspective of Self-Care Deficit theory for the care of the depressed person:
  - Nursing agency
  - Self-care agency
  - Supportive-educative role

METHOD

Lecture
Discussion

Competency 13.8

Apply the nursing process to the care of clients who are depressed.

CONTENT OUTLINE

- Review the importance of assessment for characteristics of depression during the nursing interview, including cultural elements.
- Discuss the value of intuition in detecting depression.
- Identify common nursing diagnoses associated with depression:

Hopelessness	Spiritual distress
Powerlessness	Self-care deficit
Self-esteem disturbance	Disturbed sleep pattern
Social isolation	Fatigue

- Describe interventions to assist the depressed client.

METHOD

Lecture
Discussion
Slide/transparency

Learning Experiences

Theory Application

- Use the DSM-IV-TR decision tree for affective/mood disorders to compare the different disorders noted in this chapter.
- Using an educational video, review the different behaviors and treatments for the mood-related disorders.

Individual Activities

- Have students compare and contrast the different types of depression.
- Ask students to list all the possible nursing diagnoses that apply to the diagnosis of Major Depression, Recurrent.

Group Activities

- Discussion: How should the nursing care for the person diagnosed with major depression be different from the care for a person diagnosed with a depressive episode?
- Group Seminar: The antidepressant medications

  Divide the class into three groups. Have each group develop and present a learning module on one of the following groups of medications (1) TCAs, (2) MAOIs, and (3) SSRIs. Instruct them to include the major mechanism of actions, usual method of administration, onset of initial effects, when full therapeutic effects occur, side effects, adverse reactions, and therapeutic considerations.

Clinical Activities

- Review the procedures for cognitive therapy used in treatment of depression.
- In the clinical area, review the behaviors of a client diagnosed with major depression and compare them to the DSM-IV-TR criteria for diagnoses.

Community Applications

- Identify one community-based support program for individuals who suffer from depressive disorders.
- During depression awareness month, create a health information poster to have displayed prominently at the local library, a shopping center, or a campus. Include information about the signs and resources for dealing with depression. (*Note:* The National Clearinghouse can be a ready resource for information to distribute regarding depression and the majority of clinical disorders.)

Internet Activities

- *Wings of Madness: A Depression Community* is a poignant web site, including personal accounts of depression:

  http://www.wingsofmadness.com/newsletter.htm

- The Sigma Theta Tau website has an excellent case study, "Helen Lacy and her family", which can be accessed through its online library resources:

  http://www.nursingsociety.org/education/case_studies/cases/LB001.html

NOTES

The Client Experiencing Mania

Chapter 14

Competencies

Upon completion of this chapter, the learner will be able to:

1. Define mania and state the behaviors associated with the condition.
2. Describe the cyclical relationship of mania and depression.
3. Explain the genetic and inherited nature of manic disease.
4. Describe the clinical course of mania.
5. Safely administer drugs in the treatment of mania.
6. Integrate nursing theory in assessing and understanding clients with mania.
7. Employ empathy in interactions with manic persons.
8. Use the nursing process and nursing diagnosis to plan and evaluate nursing care.

Key Terms

Bipolar Disorder	Mania
Borderline personality	Manic Episode
Continuous cycling	Rapid cycling
Cyclothymic pattern	Schizoaffective Disorder
Hypomania	Switch process

Teaching Methods and Strategies

The educator can most effectively teach about mania and bipolar disorder when clinical examples are used to highlight the behaviors and the approaches for working with the person in the manic state. Several nationally marketed videos provide excellent examples of the dynamics and the energy of the person in the manic state. In addition, the poignant stories of the lived experiences of persons who suffer from these symptoms provide powerful learning opportunities.

Lesson Plans

Topic: Mania

Competency 14.1

Define mania and state the behaviors associated with the condition.

CONTENT OUTLINE

- Define mania as an elevated, expansive, or irritable mood that interferes with functioning.
- Describe the symptoms that may accompany mania:
  - Markedly elevated mood
  - Talkativeness
  - Inflated self-esteem and grandiosity
  - Poor impulse control
  - Hypersexuality, indiscriminate sexual behavior
  - Delusions
  - Paranoia
- Describe the affective, cognitive, and behavioral manifestations of the three stages of mania.
- Describe the epidemiology of mania and bipolar disorder.
- Identify the potential role of life stress and associated disorders (dual diagnoses).

METHOD

Lecture
Slide/transparency
Review Table 14-1

Competency 14.2

Describe the cyclical relationship of mania and depression.

CONTENT OUTLINE

- Mania usually occurs with some form of depression, either separately or in close proximity.
- Switch process occurs between mania and depression.
- Number of recurrent episodes in cycles defines rapid cycling (four episodes/year) or continuous cycling.
- For a given person, length of cycle tends to be fairly constant with manic episodes typically shorter than depressive episodes.

METHOD

Lecture
Slide/transparency

Competency 14.3

Explain the genetic and inherited nature of manic disease.

CONTENT OUTLINE

- Describe genetic studies:
  - Defective gene product
  - Linkage studies
- Familial expression of affective disorders is very strong.

METHOD

Lecture
Slide/transparency
Review Figure 14-2

Competency 14.4

Describe the clinical course of mania.

CONTENT OUTLINE

- Define manic episode and describe the diagnostic criteria:
  - Distinct period of elevated mood lasting at least 1 week
  - Three symptoms persist, causing marked impairment
- Define hypomania and defining criteria:
  - Only three of the seven symptoms of mania
  - Lasts only 4 days
  - Does not cause significant disturbance in functioning
- Define bipolar disorder as a combined depression and mania most commonly in a sequential manner.
- Describe cyclothymic patterns.
- Differentiate between Bipolar I (classic) and Bipolar II Disorders.

METHOD

Lecture
Review Table 14-1

Competency 14.5

Safely administer drugs in the treatment of mania.

CONTENT OUTLINE

- Describe treatments for acute mania:
  - Benzodiazepines
  - Neuroleptics
  - Fast-acting mood stabilizer (Valproic acid)
- Describe the usefulness of maintenance pharmacological treatment.
- Describe the actions, side effects, and signs of toxicity of lithium.
- Describe the use of anticonvulsants in treating manic-depressive disorder.

METHOD

Lecture

Competency 14.6

Integrate nursing theory in assessing and understanding clients with mania.

CONTENT OUTLINE

- Describe how Parse's theory of Human Becoming can be applied to the care of the person with mania.
- Describe how Self-Care Deficit theory can be applied to the care of the person with mania.

METHOD

Lecture
Discussion

Competency 14.7

Employ empathy in interactions with manic persons.

CONTENT OUTLINE

- Describe the concept of empathy and its application to dealing with the manic person.
- Describe the behaviors most often causing a challenge to dealing empathetically with the manic person.

METHOD

Lecture
Discussion

Competency 14.8

Use the nursing process and nursing diagnosis to plan and evaluate nursing care.

CONTENT OUTLINE

- Identify important assessment questions related to the experience of mania.
- Evaluate for the presence of supporting data.
- Identify the major nursing diagnoses that apply to the manic patient regarding safety, physical, social, cognitive, and relationship needs:
  - Risk for violence
  - Disturbed sleep pattern
  - Imbalanced nutrition: less than body requirements
  - Fatigue
  - Impaired social interaction
  - Disturbed thought processes
  - Ineffective individual coping
  - Social isolation

METHOD

Lecture
Slide/transparency
Review case study/care plan

Learning Experiences

Theory Application

• Use the DSM-IV-TR decision tree for affective disorders to illustrate the differentiation between mania, the different bipolar disorders, and major depression.

• Using an educational video, review the different behaviors and treatments for manic-depressive disorder.

Individual Activities

• Have students review a standard care plan for care of the person experiencing mania.

• Direct students to identify strategies to assist the significant other/family members of the client with mania to cope.

Group Activities

• Discussion: A client decides to stop taking lithium because she misses the intensity of feelings experienced when manic. What are the pros, cons, and alternatives? What ethical dilemmas does this pose?

• Discussion: How do the behaviors of the manic individual differ from the person with borderline personality disorder? How does the nursing care differ for these individuals?

Clinical Activities

• Interview psychiatric nurses to identify the three strategies/interventions they find most useful in dealing with the manic client.

• Compare the behaviors of a client diagnosed with bipolar disorder with the DSM-IV-TR criteria.

Community Applications

• Identify one community support group for individuals with bipolar disorder.

• At the local public library, search for/identify the ready references for dealing with manic-depressive disorder.

Internet Activities

• National Institute for Mental Health reference page includes information about bipolar disorder, additional resources, and how to get more information about bipolar disorder:

http://www.thebody.com/nimh/bipolar.html

• *At Health* listing provides an excellent overview of bipolar disorder, characteristic behaviors associated with mania, epidemiology, diagnosis, and treatment:

http://www.AtHealth.com

• Home page for the National Depression and Manic-Depressive Association (NDMDA) gives information about the organization as well as multiple Internet links and resources:

http://www.ndmda.org

NOTES

The Client Who Is Suicidal

Chapter 15

Competencies

Upon completion of this chapter, the learner will be able to:

1. Explore the significance of hopelessness and loss of meaning and purpose in life.
2. Identify the conditions and circumstances that make an individual at high risk for suicide.
3. Describe a means of assessing suicide potential in a client.
4. Know the means of providing a safe environment for the suicidal patient.
5. State the psychiatric and medical conditions that significantly increase a client's suicidal risk.
6. Use theory to understand and interpret suicidal behaviors.
7. Use the nursing assessment to evaluate one's sense of meaning and purpose in life.
8. Use nursing theory to develop a therapeutic nurse-client relationship and as a framework to provide care.
9. Apply the nursing process when caring for individuals at risk for suicide.
10. Administer care to family members who have experienced the loss of a loved one through suicide.

Key Terms

Euthanasia
Suicidal ideation
Suicide
Suicide potential
Suicide survivors

Teaching Methods and Strategies

Suicide, especially among the young, is an emotional topic. An effective method of teaching about suicide and suicide prevention is to have a member of a crisis team and a family survivor discuss a case for the class. The educator must be alert to signs of distress among the students when the content is discussed. Most students will be familiar with someone who has attempted or completed suicide, and many may have personal first-hand experience. Familiarity with available resources for counseling is very important for the nurse educator in the event that a referral is needed by a student.

Lesson Plans

Topic: Suicide

Competency 15.1

Explore the significance of hopelessness and loss of meaning and purpose in life.

CONTENT OUTLINE

- Describe the atmosphere of suicide:
  - Alienation
  - Disconnectedness
  - Despair
- Identify suicide statistics:
  - Third leading cause of deaths of youths
  - Males over 65 have four times higher rate than national average
- Discuss suicide potential, suicide attempt, and suicidal ideation.

METHOD

Lecture

Competency 15.2

Identify the conditions and circumstances that make an individual at high risk for suicide.

CONTENT OUTLINE

- Discuss risk factors for suicide:
  - Age: elderly and adolescents
  - Physical illness
  - Substance abuse
  - Psychiatric diagnosis
  - Terminal, progressive disease
  - Incarceration

METHOD

Lecture
Slide/transparency

Competency 15.3

Describe a means of assessing suicide potential in a client.

CONTENT OUTLINE

- Review Table 15-1: Assessment of Suicide Potential.

- Describe at risk factors.
- Describe typical methods and lethality factor.
- Review clues to suicide:

Syndromatic	Behavioral
Verbal	Situational

- Review the common characteristics of persons attempting suicide.

METHOD

Lecture

Competency 15.4

Know the means of providing a safe environment for the suicidal patient.

CONTENT OUTLINE

- Identify primary prevention activities:
  - Access control
  - Crisis intervention
- Identify strategies to provide a safe environment:
  - Listening
  - Encouraging hospitalization
  - Restricting lethal access
  - Decreasing social isolation
  - Decreasing psychological symptoms
  - Suicide contract
- Identify the typical suicide precautions:
  - Removal of sharp objects
  - Removal of toxic substances
  - Removal of clothing that could be used for self-destruction
  - Mandate close supervision, one-to-one

METHOD

Lecture
Discussion

Competency 15.5

State the psychiatric and medical conditions that significantly increase a client's suicidal risk.

CONTENT OUTLINE

- Identify the medical conditions that have been linked with risk for suicide:

Epilepsy	Multiple sclerosis
Dementia	Brain tumor
Visual defects	Cancer

- Identify psychiatric disorders associated with suicide:

Substance abuse—drug or alcohol	Panic disorder
	Personality disorder
Depression	Obsessive-compulsive disorder
Bipolar disorder	
Conduct disorder	Mixed diagnoses
Schizophrenia	

METHOD

Lecture
Slide/transparency

Competency 15.6

Use theory to understand and interpret suicidal behaviors.

CONTENT OUTLINE

- Describe sociological factors that can explain suicide.
- Describe psychological models of suicide.
- Describe the possible biological explanations for suicide.

METHOD

Lecture

Competency 15.7

Use the nursing assessment to evaluate one's sense of meaning and purpose in life.

CONTENT OUTLINE

- Review the *Nursing Assessment of Human Spirit.*
- Review the questions in Table 15-1 and discuss them in light of one's sense of meaning.

METHOD

Lecture
Discussion
Slide/transparency

Competency 15.8

Use nursing theory to develop a therapeutic nurse-client relationship and as a framework to provide care.

CONTENT OUTLINE

- Using Peplau's theory, identify the major needs of the suicidal individual that can be met via the nurse-patient relationship:
  - Be cared about and loved
  - Maintain self-esteem
  - Sense some control over life
  - Sense interpersonal support
- Identify what the nurse provides:
  - Time
  - Support
  - Boundaries
  - Interpersonal interactions
  - Resources to meet needs
  - Clarification

METHOD

Discussion

Competency 15.9

Apply the nursing process when caring for individuals at risk for suicide.

CONTENT OUTLINE

- Review risk assessment.
- Identify major nursing diagnoses:
  - Helplessness
  - Powerlessness
  - Spiritual distress
- Review primary, secondary, and tertiary prevention measures.

METHOD

Lecture
Discussion

Competency 15.10

Administer care to family members who have experienced the loss of a loved one through suicide.

CONTENT OUTLINE

- Review the nursing information on how to help survivors.
- Discuss possible risk factors for survivors.
- Identify the role of self-help groups and bereavement networks.

METHOD

Lecture
Discussion

Learning Experiences

Theory Application

- Review the psychological theories presented in Unit 1 and apply them to the case study of Penny.
- How would a nurse using the nursing theories of Orem or Rogers approach the care of the suicidal person?

Individual Activities

- Ask students to reflect on the questions that this chapter has brought to their minds about suicide.
- In their journals, have students indicate the feelings they experience when reading the excerpt in the section titled Adolescents and Young Adults.

Group Activities

- Discussion: Thoughts on assisted suicide
- Project: Develop a pamphlet about suicide, its relationship to physical diagnoses, and preventive tips for distribution to general hospital staff.

Clinical Activities

- The next time they are on the clinical unit, direct students to walk around and notice the things that could pose potential hazards for a suicidal client.
- Discuss with nursing staff their experiences with suicidal clients and their reactions to any situation where a client has committed suicide.

Community Applications

- Find the suicide hotline number for your community.
- Assist a local high school to develop an assembly to present the topic or listen to a guest speaker about suicide prevention and how to help a friend in need.

Internet Activities

- A variety of topics relating to suicide can be found on psycom.net, e.g., scientific study of brain chemistry as it relates to markers for suicide:

  http://www.psycom.net/depression.central.suicide.html
- This site has a direct personal message of caring, coping suggestions, and information about suicide and suicide prevention:

  http://www.metanoia.org
- The role of serotonin and its usefulness as a marker for intervention before suicide are described on this web site:

  http://www.mhsource.com/edu/psytimes/p950907.html

NOTES

The Client Who Abuses Chemical Substances

Chapter 16

Competencies

Upon completion of this chapter, the learner will be able to:

1. Describe the widespread nature of substance abuse in historical and modern times.
2. List the types of substances open to misuse and abuse.
3. Define and differentiate between the terms *tolerance, withdrawal, dependence, craving,* and *addiction.*
4. Identify the effects, withdrawal symptoms, patterns of abuse, and means of treatment for nicotine, alcohol, cocaine, and opiate abuse.
5. Explain the philosophy and treatment approach of Alcoholics Anonymous and 12-step programs.
6. Explain the relationship of chemical abuse and family dysfunction.
7. Explain the dynamics of codependency.
8. Employ nursing theory and diagnoses to plan care for the individual and family unit where chemical abuse is occurring.

Key Terms

Addiction	Drug use
Alcoholism	Substance abuse
Codependence	Tolerance
Craving	Withdrawal
Drug dependence	

Teaching Methods and Strategies

There are more pages in the DSM-IV-TR devoted to substance-related disorders than any other group of psychiatric disorders. The problems of substance abuse influence every specialty area of health care. As such, the nurse has a strong role in prevention, case identification, and intervention. It is suggested that the educator supplement the information in this chapter with specific information from the DSM-IV-TR and references about psychopharmacology. The content of this chapter provides an overview of some of the factors related to the treatment of substance abuse. The complexity of these disorders requires that nurses learn this information and much more to be effective in providing care to individuals who suffer from substance abuse disorders.

Lesson Plans

Topic: Abuse of Chemical Substances

Competency 16.1

Describe the widespread nature of substance abuse in historical and modern times.

CONTENT OUTLINE

- Identify some historical references to substance use and abuse.
- Describe some efforts that have been implemented in an effort to control substance abuse:
  - Tobacco
  - Alcohol
  - Harrison Act

METHOD

Lecture

Competency 16.2

List the types of substances open to misuse and abuse.

CONTENT OUTLINE

- Discuss the misuse and abuse of psychoactive substances.
- Identify commonly abused substances:
  - Nicotine
  - Alcohol
  - Cocaine
  - Opiates, e.g., heroine
  - Hallucinogens
  - Inhalants
  - Marijuana

METHOD

Slide/transparency

Competency 16.3

Define and differentiate between the terms *tolerance, withdrawal, dependence, craving,* and *addiction.*

CONTENT OUTLINE

- Review the definitions of tolerance, dependence, and addiction.
- Describe the phenomenon of craving.
- Define withdrawal in terms of the effects of a substance.

METHOD

Lecture
Discussion

Competency 16.4

Identify the effects, withdrawal symptoms, patterns of abuse, and means of treatment for nicotine, alcohol, cocaine, and opiate abuse.

CONTENT OUTLINE

- Describe the effects, symptoms of withdrawal, and treatment approaches for nicotine:

  Effects and patterns: Subjective relaxation with excitement, improved motor performance, decreased appetite (especially females); so physically and psychologically addicting there is little distinction between abuse and dependence

  Withdrawal: Anxiety, mood change, frustration, anger, irritability, restlessness, fatigue, difficulty concentrating, hunger, EEG alterations, sweating

  Treatment: Nicotine replacement gums, patches initially; psychological and behavioral programs to recognize potential relapse situations and behavior management approaches; community education

- Describe the effects, symptoms of withdrawal, and treatment approaches for alcohol:

  Effects and patterns: Disinhibition, talkativeness, incoordination, irritability, combativeness, slurred speech, drowsiness, impaired cognitive functioning; chronic effects cause damage to cardiovascular, gastrointestinal, endocrine, reproductive, and neurological systems; lead to social and psychological impairment and disorders; abuse, dependence, alcoholism—phases of drinking behavior

  Withdrawal: Sweating, rapid pulse, tremors, hallucinations, sleep disorder, nausea, vomiting, agitation, delirium

  Treatment: Detoxification, benzodiazepines, naltrexane, counseling, Alcoholics Anonymous/12-step programs, screening, education, and BRIEF intervention.

- Describe the effects, symptoms of withdrawal, and treatment approaches for cocaine:

  Effects and patterns: Stimulates brain's reward centers, euphoria, increased sense of energy, enhanced mental acuity, increased sensory awareness, decreased appetite, increased anxiety and suspiciousness, decreased need for sleep, increased self-confidence, egocentricity, delusions; tolerance is common, craving intense

  Withdrawal: Fatigue, vivid nightmares, sleep disturbance, increased appetite, psychomotor changes, cravings, post-intoxication "crash," depression

  Treatment: Counseling, 12-step programs, treating depression, lifestyle modification

- Describe the effects, symptoms of withdrawal, and treatment approaches for opiate substances:

  Effects and patterns: Diminished perception of pain, initial rush of pleasure, sense of comfort, contentment, slowed down body functions; tolerance, dependence

  Withdrawal: Depression, restlessness, nausea, vomiting, muscle aches, tearing, dilated pupils, sweating, yawning, diarrhea, fever, insomnia

  Treatment: Complex combination of physical, psychological, and social factors, detoxification, pharmacological agents to ease detoxification

- Describe the effects, symptoms of withdrawal, and treatment approaches for hallucinogen substances:

  Effects and patterns: Euphoria, heightened sensory perception, dream state, sense of invincibility, may engage in dangerous behaviors while under the influence; tolerance develops quickly but rarely does dependence develop

  Withdrawal: None

  Treatment: Abstinence, education

METHOD

Lecture
Discussion
Group seminar

Competency 16.5

Explain the philosophy and treatment approach of Alcoholics Anonymous and 12-step programs.

CONTENT OUTLINE

- Describe the philosophy of AA.
- Review the 12-step approach to dealing with addictions.
- Discuss the element of group support and identification provided by self-help approaches to recovery.

METHOD

Lecture
Discussion

Competency 16.6

Explain the relationship of chemical abuse and family dysfunction.

CONTENT OUTLINE

- Describe substance abuse as a social problem.
- Discuss interrupted family processes and dynamics.
- Discuss the impact of substance abuse on the family.

METHOD

Lecture
Discussion

Competency 16.7

Explain the dynamics of codependency.

CONTENT OUTLINE

- Define codependency.
- Discuss the dynamics of codependent behaviors.
- Identify self-help groups that can assist family members to deal with substance use and codependency issues.

METHOD

Lecture

Competency 16.8

Employ nursing theory and diagnoses to plan care for the individual and family unit where chemical abuse is occurring.

CONTENT OUTLINE

- Describe the application of interpersonal nursing theory to guide nursing care.
- Identify the importance of the concepts of caring, support, and self-responsibility.
- Identify some nursing diagnoses used for clients with substance abuse disorders:
  - Ineffective individual coping
  - Interrupted family processes
  - Hopelessness

METHOD

Lecture
Slide/transparency

Learning Experiences

Theory Application

- Review the CAGE questionnaire and how the questions reflect a theoretical perspective about alcoholism.
- Discuss, in depth, the phases of drinking described in Table 16-3 and apply them to a case example.

Individual Activities

- Have students attend at least one 12-step recovery meeting to better understand this resource for the person who has a diagnosis of substance abuse.
- Ask students to create a list of all the potential nursing diagnoses that might apply to an individual with the diagnosis of substance abuse.
- In their journals, have students describe their thoughts on each of the following statements:
  1. Like diabetes, substance abuse is a disability.
  2. Like schizophrenia, substance abuse is a mental disability.

Group Activities

- Awareness Heightening Activity: Its in black and white

  Assign the students to two groups. Group 1 is to go get a newspaper from a rural area. Group 2 is to get a newspaper from an urban area. As a group, they are to read every page of their group's newspaper, identify the items that deal with substance abuse in some form, and make a listing. At the next class, the lists are compared and discussed.

- Project: Substances of abuse information

  Divide the class into four groups. Each group is to develop a two-page chart of the substances, effects, symptoms of overdose, withdrawal symptoms, and means of treatment of one of the following categories: stimulants, depressants, opiates, and hallucinogens.

Clinical Activities

- In the DSM-IV-TR, read the chapter on substance-related disorders to gain a better understanding of these disorders.
- Investigate what percentage of psychiatric admissions for acute care are related to substance abuse and what percentage of emergency department cases involve substance abuse.

Community Applications

- Visit a bookstore in your neighborhood and note the number of self-help books that are written about substance abuse, addictions, recovery, codependency, and the like.
- Get involved in a community health fair with a booth about substance abuse, treatment resources, and information for distribution.

Internet Activities

- The home page for the National Institutes on Drug Abuse contains information about the institutes as well as an extensive number of links:

  http://www.nida.nih.gov

- The Substance Abuse and Mental Health Services Administration (DHHS) web page provides information, links, and an overview of substance abuse prevention initiatives:

  http://www.samhsa.gov/csap

- The URL for the National Clearinghouse for Alcohol and Drug Information (NCADI):

  http://www.health.org/aboutn.htm

- The home page for the World Service Organization of Cocaine Anonymous, which includes information about the self-help organization, a self-test for cocaine addiction, public information, and more, can be reached via:

  http://www.ca.org

NOTES

The Client with a Personality Disorder

Chapter 17

Competencies

Upon completion of this chapter, the learner will be able to:

1. Define personality, personality trait, and personality disorder.
2. Differentiate between a person with eccentric personality traits and a person with a personality disorder.
3. Identify characteristics of specific personality disorders.
4. Describe how early childhood influences can affect personality development.
5. Use nursing theory to understand a client with a personality disorder and to plan appropriate nursing interventions.

Key Terms

Antisocial Personality Disorder
Avoidant Personality Disorder
Borderline Personality Disorder
Dependent Personality Disorder
Histrionic Personality Disorder
Narcissistic Personality Disorder
Obsessive-Compulsive Personality Disorder
Paranoid Personality Disorder
Passive-Aggressive Personality Disorder
Personality
Personality disorder
Personality traits
Schizoid Personality Disorder
Schizotypal Personality Disorder

Teaching Methods and Strategies

The educator is always challenged to explain the distinct differences between personality disorders as Axis II diagnoses and the Axis I diagnoses that seem so similar. In this chapter, the authors have provided several sets of boxed information considering these similarities and differences.

Following the DSM-IV-TR approach to clusters of personality disorders based on characteristics, the educator can compare and contrast the clusters quite easily. Also, the essential features of each of the personality disorders have been pulled out so the student has ready references.

The nursing care for individuals with personality disorders follows the symptoms displayed in each individual case. However, it is imperative to share with the student the need to understand that the behaviors that the person displays occur from some sense of self-preservation: although at times very aggravating and frustrating, the behaviors are inherent in the patient's personality.

Lesson Plans

Topic: Personality Disorders

Competency 17.1

Define personality, personality trait, and personality disorder.

CONTENT OUTLINE

- Describe personality as the sum total of the habitual patterns and qualities of the individual.
- Define personality traits as those individual qualities that make a person unique.
- Define personality disorder (as per DSM-IV-TR) as an enduring, pervasive, persistent, and inflexible pattern of behaviors and inner experiences that differ markedly from cultural expectations, with onset in adolescence or early adulthood, stable over time, and causing distress or impairment.

METHOD

Lecture

Competency 17.2

Differentiate between a person with eccentric personality traits and a person with a personality disorder.

CONTENT OUTLINE

- Discuss how eccentricity differs from the definition of personality disorder (above).

METHOD

Lecture
Discussion

Competency 17.3

Identify characteristics of specific personality disorders.

CONTENT OUTLINE

- Identify the three clusters of personality disorders:
  - Dramatic and emotional
    - Borderline Personality Disorder
    - Narcissistic Personality Disorder
    - Histrionic Personality Disorder
    - Antisocial Personality Disorder
  - Odd and eccentric
    - Schizoid Personality Disorder
    - Schizotypal Personality Disorder
    - Paranoid Personality Disorder
  - Anxiety and fear based
    - Obsessive-Compulsive Personality Disorder
    - Avoidant Personality Disorder
    - Dependent Personality Disorder
- Describe the essential features of Borderline Personality Disorder.
- Describe the essential features of Narcissistic Personality Disorder.
- Describe the essential features of Histrionic Personality Disorder.
- Describe the essential features of Antisocial Personality Disorder.
- Describe the essential features of Schizoid Personality Disorder.
- Describe the essential features of Schizotypal Personality Disorder.
- Describe the essential features of Paranoid Personality Disorder.
- Describe the essential features of Obsessive-Compulsive Personality Disorder.
- Describe the essential features of Avoidant Personality Disorder.
- Describe the essential features of Dependent Personality Disorder.

METHOD

Slide/transparency of boxed information about essential features
Review Table 17-1

Competency 17.4

Describe how early childhood influences can affect personality development.

CONTENT OUTLINE

- Discuss possible environmental factors that contribute to development of personality disorders.
- Discuss family developmental etiological factors in the development of personality disorders.

METHOD

Lecture
Discussion

Competency 17.5

Use nursing theory to understand a client with a personality disorder and to plan appropriate nursing interventions.

CONTENT OUTLINE

- Apply Erickson's theory of modeling and role modeling to explore personality disorders.
- Apply Roger's theory of unitary human beings to understand personality disorders.
- Review Table 17-2, Listing of Nursing Diagnoses, for diagnoses that apply to individuals experiencing personality disorders.
- Review Table 17-3, Nursing Interventions and Rationale, for care of clients with personality disorders.

METHOD

Lecture
Discussion
Slide/transparency

Learning Experiences

Theory Application

- Compare the nursing approaches of Peplau, Rogers, and Erickson in caring for the client with a diagnosis of personality disorder.
- Discuss developmental theories and personality disorders.

Individual Activities

- In their journals, have students describe their reactions to the excerpt titled *Annie*.
- Based on the behaviors described in *Annie*, direct students to develop a plan of care for this client with Borderline Personality Disorder.

Group Activities

- Discussion: As a group, discuss the differences between paranoid schizophrenia and Paranoid Personality Disorder.
- Discussion: As a group, discuss the differences between schizophrenia, Schizoid Personality Disorder, and Schizotypal Personality Disorder.

Clinical Activities

- Discuss with psychiatric nurses their reactions to dealing with clients with personality disorders.
- Discuss with the attending psychiatrist: (1) the average number of clients who present with Axis II diagnoses in any given month; (2) the intensity of therapy required by such a client; and (3) perspective on prognosis.

Community Applications

- Where in the community might you meet a person with Histrionic Personality Disorder?
- In your community, what services or programs tend to deal with individuals with Antisocial Personality Disorder?

Internet Activities

- At this mentalhealth.com URL, the menu allows you to review descriptions of the personality disorders:

  http://www.mentalhealth.com

NOTES

The Client Experiencing a Psychosomatic Illness

Chapter 18

Competencies

Upon completion of this chapter, the learner will be able to:

1. Define somatoform disorders, and distinguish among Somatization Disorder, Hypochondriasis, and Conversion Disorder.
2. Define Factitious Disorder (Munchausen's Syndrome) and Munchausen's Syndrome by Proxy.
3. Describe the presenting characteristics of an individual with Somatization Disorder who comes to an acute-care clinic for diagnosis and treatment.
4. Distinguish between Hypochondriasis and Anxiety Disorder.
5. Present the major theoretical explanations for Hypochondriasis (psychoanalytical, behavioral, and biological).
6. Describe principles for the effective treatment of Hypochondriasis.
7. Provide an explanation for treatment of Conversion Disorder through direct explanation of the underlying conflict.
8. Differentiate between Factitious Disorder and malingering.
9. Utilize the nursing process and nursing theory to plan care for clients experiencing psychosomatic illness.
10. Use techniques of introspection and self-reflection to examine your own feelings with regard to clients whose physical complaints are a result of psychiatric illness.

Key Terms

Conversion Disorder
Factitious Disorder
Hypochondriasis
Malingering
Munchausen's Syndrome
Munchausen's Syndrome by Proxy
Somatization Disorder
Somatoform Disorder

Teaching Methods and Strategies

The disorders presented in this chapter are representative of the diagnostic category of psychosomatic illness. The diagnostic criteria are provided in a boxed format that allows ready access for comparison and for use as transparencies. Because the psychosomatic illnesses are relatively rare, the educator may wish to spend only a brief time reviewing the information.

Lesson Plans

Topic: Psychosomatic Illness

Competency 18.1

Define somatoform disorders, and distinguish among Somatization Disorder, Hypochondriasis, and Conversion Disorder.

CONTENT OUTLINE

- Describe the somatoform disorders as a group of psychological conditions that manifest in physical symptoms that suggest a general medical condition, but careful clinical evaluation fails to find any evidence of physical disorder to explain the complaints.
- Define somatization disorder as multiple physical complaints without apparent physiological cause.
- Describe hypochondriasis as a condition marked by preoccupation with fear of a serious disease based on misinterpretation of bodily symptoms and functions.
- Describe Conversion Disorder as a condition where the person exhibits physical symptoms that cannot be explained by neurological or medical conditions.

METHOD

Lecture

Competency 18.2

Define Factitious Disorder (Munchausen's Syndrome) and Munchausen's Syndrome by Proxy.

CONTENT OUTLINE

- Define Factitious Disorder, also known as Munchausen's Syndrome, as a condition marked by physical or psychological symptoms that are intentionally produced to gain attention.
- Describe Munchausen's Syndrome by Proxy as a form of child abuse in which the caregiver falsely reports a child's illness resulting in unnecessary medical treatment.

- Note that the actual prevalence is unknown and factors leading to Factitious Disorder are unclear.
- The nature of this disorder makes it almost impossible to treat.

METHOD

Lecture

Competency 18.3

Describe the presenting characteristics of an individual with Somatization Disorder who comes to an acute-care clinic for diagnosis and treatment.

CONTENT OUTLINE

- Describe the diagnostic criteria for somatization disorder.
- Describe epidemiological information about somatization disorder.
    - Relatively rare (0.13%)
    - Women ten times greater occurrence
    - Tends to occur in families, especially families where antisocial personality disorder can be diagnosed
    - Exact cause is unknown: Both heredity and environment contribute to development of somatization disorder
- Describe the three therapeutic goals of psychotherapy with the patient diagnosed with somatization disorder:
    - Establishing a therapeutic alliance
    - Educating client regarding manifestations
    - Providing consistent reassurance
- Identify other considerations of treatment:
    - Diagnosis remains tentative
    - Appropriate vigilance in the face of seemingly endless subjective complaints
    - Caretaker fatigue

METHOD

Lecture

Competency 18.4

Distinguish between Hypochondriasis and Anxiety Disorder.

CONTENT OUTLINE

- Define Hypochondriasis as preoccupation with fear of having a serious disease.
- Describe the diagnostic criteria for Hypochondriasis.
- Compare the criteria for Hypochondriasis with those for Anxiety Disorder.

METHOD

Lecture

Competency 18.5

Present the major theoretical explanations for Hypochondriasis (psychoanalytical, behavioral, and biological).

CONTENT OUTLINE

- Describe the psychoanalytical perspective of Hypochondriasis—repressed anger and hostility.
- Describe the behavioral perspective of Hypochondriasis—learned behavior that is rewarded, reinforced.
- Describe the biological perspective of Hypochondriasis—individual excessive sensitivity to normal bodily sensations.

METHOD

Lecture

Competency 18.6

Describe principles for the effective treatment of Hypochondriasis.

CONTENT OUTLINE

- A physical exam and reassurance should precede any treatment and be repeated during treatment process, especially if a new symptom appears.
- Treat any concurrent psychiatric condition as indicated.
- Educate the client about the nature of Hypochondriasis. Individual must understand how perception of bodily sensations leads to overemphasis on illness. Psychotherapy focuses on learning to ignore symptoms through retraining.

METHOD

Lecture
Discussion
Review boxed information

Competency 18.7

Provide an explanation for treatment of Conversion Disorder through direct explanation of the underlying conflict.

CONTENT OUTLINE

- Define Conversion Disorder.
- Identify the diagnostic criteria for Conversion Disorder.
- Identify the two central features of Conversion Disorder:
    1. No medical condition explains the symptoms.
    2. Symptoms occur as a result of psychological factors.

METHOD

Lecture
Review boxed information, Diagnostic Criteria

Competency 18.8

Differentiate between Factitious Disorder and malingering.

CONTENT OUTLINE

- Define malingering.

- Differentiate between feigned symptoms for the purpose of achieving some objective goal (e.g., financial compensation) noted in malingering versus the complex mixture of truth and falsehoods with dramatic embellishment and subjective gains noted with factitious disorders.

METHOD

Lecture

Competency 18.9

Utilize the nursing process and nursing theory to plan care for clients experiencing psychosomatic illness.

CONTENT OUTLINE

- Apply Watson's theory of human caring to plan care for the person experiencing psychosomatic illness:
  - Strive for caring interpersonal relationship
  - Give care without demands for engaging
- Apply Erickson's modeling and role modeling theory to plan care for the person experiencing psychosomatic illness:
  - Focus on understanding the client's subjective experience
  - Listen
  - Strive to build a trusting nurse-client relationship
- Identify nursing diagnoses that may be applicable to planning care for the client with a psychosomatic diagnosis:
  - Disturbed body image
  - Disturbed self-esteem
  - Ineffective individual coping
  - Powerlessness
  - Social isolation

METHOD

Lecture
Discussion
Slide/transparency

Competency 18.10

Use techniques of introspection and self-reflection to examine your own feelings with regard to clients whose physical complaints are a result of psychiatric illness.

CONTENT OUTLINE

- Review questions to ask self as the caregiver:
  - Does the client need a nurse?
  - Do I believe the person?
  - Can the mental disorder take precedence over the physical problems?
  - How do I feel when the client does not want to get well?
- Discuss the role of compassion in caring for the client with a psychosomatic disorder.

METHOD

Lecture
Discussion

Learning Experiences

Theory Application

- Review the DSM-IV-TR information regarding psychosomatic disorders.
- Discuss the potential for using behavioral and cognitive frameworks in dealing with the person with a psychosomatic disorder.

Individual Activities

- Have students review the list of NANDA diagnoses and identify all the possible nursing diagnoses that apply to the person diagnosed with Hypochondriasis.
- In their journals, direct students to reflect on their own reactions to the questions posed for the nurse about caring for the person with a somatoform disorder.

Group Activities

- Discussion: Ethical issues associated with care of the person with Munchausen's Syndrome
- Seminar: Application of nursing theory

  Assign students to apply a particular nurse theorist's framework to the planning of care for a client with Conversion Disorder. The plans are then presented in a seminar and discussed as a group.

Clinical Activities

- Review the clinical procedures and plans of care for a person diagnosed with a somatoform disorder.
- Discuss with two staff nurses their perspectives about Munchausen's Syndrome by Proxy.

Community Applications

- Identify one community-based support group for individuals with somatoform disorders.

Internet Activities

- The URL for the home page of the American Psychosomatic Society also links to the contents of the newsletter of the Society:

  http://www.psychosomatic.org

NOTES

The Client with Disorders of Self-Regulation: Sleep Disorders, Eating Disorders, Sexual Disorders

Chapter 19

Competencies

Upon completion of this chapter, the learner will be able to:

1. Describe normal sleep cycles and changes in sleep cycles expected in aging.
2. Assess clients for the presence of Insomnia.
3. Provide a sleep hygiene regimen for clients with disturbed sleep.
4. Define Primary Hypersomnia.
5. Identify parasomnias and provide appropriate nursing interventions and support.
6. Assess clients for the presence of Bulimia and Anorexia Nervosa.
7. Plan nursing care for clients with eating disorders, including nutritional rehabilitation, psychotherapy, maintenance, and follow-up care.
8. Assess clients for altered sexuality, sexual dysfunction, and sexual disorders.
9. Utilize nursing theory and nursing process in planning and providing care for clients with disorders of regulation.

Key Terms

Anorexia Nervosa
Bulimia Nervosa
Cataplexy
Dyssomnia
Exhibitionism
Fetishism
Frotteurism
Gender dysphoria
Gender identity
Gender Identity Disorder
Gender role
Hypoactive Sexual Desire Disorder
Insomnia
Narcolepsy
Nightmare
Normal sexual behavior
Paraphilia
Parasomnia
Pedophilia
Primary Hypersomnia
Primary Insomnia
Sexual dysfunction
Sexual masochism
Sexual sadism
Sleep hygiene
Sleep latency
Sleep paralysis
Sleep terrors
Sleepwalking
Transvestic fetishism
Voyeurism

Teaching Methods and Strategies

The information in this chapter covers three separate DSM-IV-TR categories of disorders. The common theme among the topics is dysregulation. The educator may opt to use the theme as a unifying element or to present the separate disorders and then link them via the theme.

Each of the three topics of this chapter has much more extensive and specialized information than is possible to present in this textbook. It will be important to guide students in understanding that these are subspecialty areas that can be independently explored.

Lesson Plans

Topic: Disorders of Self-Regulation

Competency 19.1

Describe normal sleep cycles and changes in sleep cycles expected in aging.

CONTENT OUTLINE

- Identify the stages of sleep.
- Describe the typical sleep cycle of the adult.
- Identify how the sleep cycle changes with aging.

METHOD

Lecture
Discussion
Slide/transparency

Competency 19.2

Assess clients for the presence of insomnia.

CONTENT OUTLINE

- Define insomnia as difficulty in initiating or maintaining sleep.
- Review the boxed questions for assessment of sleep patterns.

METHOD

Lecture
Slide/transparency

Competency 19.3

Provide a sleep hygiene regimen for clients with disturbed sleep.

CONTENT OUTLINE

- Define sleep hygiene as specific activities that assist in achieving restful sleep.
- Identify techniques of sleep hygiene:
  - Restrict bed and bedroom for sleep
  - Arise at the same time each day regardless of when went to bed
  - Exercise daily, preferably late afternoon
  - Keep room quiet, dark, and at a comfortable temperature
  - Avoid daytime napping
  - Avoid caffeine and alcohol in evening
  - Position clock so it cannot be seen
  - If possible, sometimes break the cycle of insomnia by staying awake for an entire night

METHOD

Lecture
Slide/transparency

Competency 19.4

Define Primary Hypersomnia.

CONTENT OUTLINE

- Define Primary Hypersomnia as daytime sleepiness for which there is no external or physiological explanation.
- Identify characteristics of hypersomnia:
  - Decreased sleep latency
  - Lack of REM sleep
- Differentiate between Primary Hypersomnia and Narcolepsy:
  - Irresistible need for brief episodes of sleep
  - Sleep paralysis
  - Cataplexy

METHOD

Lecture

Competency 19.5

Identify parasomnias and provide appropriate nursing interventions and support.

CONTENT OUTLINE

- Identify three common parasomnias: nightmares, sleep terrors, and sleepwalking.
- Describe the characteristics of each parasomnia:
  - *Nightmare:* Exceedingly vivid dreams of frightening content; on awakening have good recall of content and recall accompanied by persistent anxiety
  - *Sleep terrors:* No recall of the sleep-related event; rouse suddenly from sleep with cry or scream; sit up in bed in terror (sweaty, dilated pupils, tachypneic, tachycardic); physical activity of fighting or striking out; cannot be awakened; only fragmentary recall or no memory of physical activity of fighting
  - *Sleepwalking:* Pattern of getting out of bed, not fully conscious; difficult to arouse and if awakened very confused, no recall of events
- Describe nursing interventions for nursing diagnosis of Disturbed Sleep Pattern:
  - Reassurance
  - Sympathetic interviewing and counseling
  - Sleep pattern assessment
  - Ensure protection and security

METHOD

Lecture
Case example

Competency 19.6

Assess clients for the presence of Bulimia and Anorexia Nervosa.

CONTENT OUTLINE

- Describe the characteristics associated with bulimia:
  - Preoccupation with weight and body appearance
  - Binging and lack of control
  - Fasting, purging, laxative abuse to achieve control and restrict weight gain
  - Consequential erosion of tooth enamel, stones in the salivary glands, esophageal veracies, electrolyte disturbances
  - Depression
  - Substance abuse to control appetite and weight
- Review screening questions for bulimia (satisfied with eating pattern, eat in secret).
- Describe the characteristics associated with anorexia:
  - Profound disturbance in body image
  - Starvation, dieting, exercising
  - Profound body changes
  - Emaciation
  - Amenorrhea
  - Dry skin
  - Lanugo
  - Cardiac dysrhythmia, syncope, bradycardia
  - Intense fear of gaining weight
  - Distorted appraisal of body size and shape
- Identify proposed causative factors for anorexia:
  - Desire to suppress adult sexual development and responsibility
  - Disordered family structure and function
  - Failed perfectionist tendencies so strive to control eating

Poor self-esteem, distorted body image, and inability to process interoceptive stimuli such as being hungry and feeling full

METHOD

Lecture
Discussion

Competency 19.7

Plan nursing care for clients with eating disorders, including nutritional rehabilitation, psychotherapy, maintenance, and follow-up care.

CONTENT OUTLINE

- Identify treatments for eating disorders:
  - Antidepressant pharmacotherapy
  - Cognitive-behavioral therapy
  - Anxiolytics for OCD
- Identify common nursing diagnoses for clients with eating disorders:
  - Imbalanced nutrition
  - Disturbed body image
  - Low self-esteem
  - Social isolation
  - Ineffective health maintenance
  - Powerlessness
- Discuss prioritization of treatment:
  - Physiological stability
  - Nutritional rehabilitation (halt starvation, establish appropriate eating pattern, monitor intake, weight gain)
  - Psychotherapy (individual, group, support)
  - Maintenance (self-monitoring, internal strategies developed, stress management)

METHOD

Lecture
Discussion
Slide/transparency

Competency 19.8

Assess clients for altered sexuality, sexual dysfunction, and sexual disorders.

CONTENT OUTLINE

- Identify the three topics to assess in a sexual history:
  - Sexual functioning
  - Fantasies, thoughts, and behaviors
  - Preferences
- Describe disorders of sexual functioning:
  - Disorders of desire
  - Hypoactive sexual desire disorder
  - Premature ejaculation
- Describe paraphilias, disorders of sexual thought, fantasy, or behavior:
  - Exhibitionism
  - Transvestic fetishism
  - Sexual sadism
  - Sexual masochism
  - Pedophilia
  - Frotteurism
  - Voyeurism
- Describe gender identity disorder.
- Identify nursing diagnoses for care of the client with sexual disorders:
  - Ineffective sexuality patterns
  - Disturbed self-esteem
  - Ineffective individual coping
  - Impaired social interaction
  - Anxiety

METHOD

Lecture
Slide/transparency
Review boxed information of defining characteristics

Competency 19.9

Utilize nursing theory and nursing process in planning and providing care for clients with disorders of regulation.

CONTENT OUTLINE

- Apply Watson's theory of human care to planning for the person with disorders of regulation:
  - Acceptance
  - Positive regard
  - Interpersonal relationship

METHOD

Discussion

Learning Experiences

Theory Application

- Review the DSM-IV-TR information and diagnostic criteria for the different sexual disorders.
- Using an educational video, review the different behaviors and treatment approaches for eating disorders.

Individual Activities

- In their journals, have students discuss their perspectives about working with a client with Anorexia Nervosa.
- Direct students to review a standard care plan for a client with Primary Insomnia.

Group Activities

- Discussion: In reality, how do gender and sexual orientation play a role in care provided? How is this affected when the client has a sexual disorder?

• Survey: Develop a series of questions to determine the extent of sleep disruptions experienced by psychiatric clients and the behavioral descriptions. Then compare these with the diagnostic criteria for sleep disorders.

Clinical Activities

• Visit a sleep disorders center.

• Develop a handout about medications that can be useful in treating disorders of regulation. Share this with clinical unit staff.

Community Applications

• At a health fair, have a booth with information about eating disorders, treatments, and resources.

• Attend a community-based meeting of Overeaters Anonymous.

Internet Activities

• This guide to sleep disorders includes links for information about insomnia, narcolepsy, sleep apnea, and restless leg syndrome:

http://www.sleepnet.com/disorder.htm

• Readings, resources, and a discussion zone where reactions to personal experiences and reflections may be found in this site for *Self-Help* and *Psychology* magazines:

http://cybertowers.com/selfhelp/articles/eating/nih/index.html

• American Anorexia/Bulimia Association, Inc. has a web site with information and resources for those who suffer, their family, friends, and professionals:

http://www.aabainc.org

• Information about paraphilias can be located at:

http://www.athealth.com/consumer/disorders/paraphilias.html

Unit

3

Special Populations

The six chapters in Unit 3 focus on the needs and nursing care perspectives for special populations. Populations may be special by virtue of diagnosis, age, social circumstance, and other factors.

The challenge of caring for both the emotional and physical needs is reviewed in Chapter 20. The psychiatric nursing care of the "forgotten populations," the homeless and the incarcerated, is the focus of Chapter 21. Although many of these individuals actually have Axis I diagnoses, they are the focus of the social and judicial systems of society.

In addition, psychiatric nursing concerns vary with specific age groups. Chapters 22, 23, and 24 highlight specifics of psychiatric nursing care for the child, the adolescent, and the elderly.

The last chapter in this unit deals with the needs of survivors of violence and abuse. The topics in this chapter include neglect, child abuse, rape, domestic violence, and elder abuse.

NOTES

The Physically Ill Client Experiencing Emotional Distress

Chapter 20

Competencies

Upon completion of this chapter, the learner will be able to:

1. Identify those situations where a physical illness produces emotional stress to the point where a client may present with psychological symptoms.
2. Describe the common reactions clients have to cancer, heart disease, chronic pain, and neurological disorders that require attention to mental health and psychological adjustments.
3. Describe the role of the psychiatric liaison nurse.
4. Describe the role of the community mental health nurse in home care settings.
5. Describe the emerging field of body-mind medicine and its effects on holistic nursing care.
6. Utilize nursing theory to complete holistic nursing assessments and provide interventions in situations where the client is facing both physical and psychiatric symptoms.

Key Terms

Liaison psychiatric nursing
Liaison psychiatry
Mind modulation

Teaching Methods and Strategies

This chapter offers numerous case examples of the complex emotional elements of physical illness. The examples can serve as a vehicle to discuss the importance of psychiatric nursing for these clients. This is also a point where experiences from other courses can be linked with the psychiatric information from earlier chapters. As such, a discussion format can further facilitate the learning process.

Lesson Plans

Topic: Physical Illness and Emotional Distress

Competency 20.1

Identify those situations where a physical illness produces emotional stress to the point where a client may present with psychological symptoms.

CONTENT OUTLINE

- Physical conditions provoke situations that are emotionally laden:
  - Threaten autonomy
  - Loss of livelihood
  - Risk of death
  - Interference with social relationships
  - Threaten self-image and self-esteem
  - Require dramatic lifestyle adjustments
  - Loss of motor functioning
  - Forced dependence
- Identify some conditions that have a strong concomitant emotional component:

Cancer	Arthritis
Heart attack	Paralysis
Blindness	Multiple sclerosis

METHOD

Lecture
Discussion

Competency 20.2

Describe the common reactions clients have to cancer, heart disease, chronic pain, and neurological disorders that require attention to mental health and psychological adjustments.

CONTENT OUTLINE

- Describe the grief response.
- Describe the symptoms of depression.
- Describe the responses to the aforementioned illnesses:

Hopelessness	Loss of identity	Anger
Sense of failure	Fatigue	Guilt
Social isolation	Fear	Grief
Loss of meaning	Anxiety	Depression

METHOD

Lecture
Discussion

Competency 20.3

Describe the role of the psychiatric liaison nurse.

CONTENT OUTLINE

- Discuss the need for the liaison nurse to provide nonpsychiatric health care providers with consultation.
- Review the goals of psychiatric liaison nursing.

METHOD
Lecture
Discussion

Competency 20.4

Describe the role of the community mental health nurse in home care settings.

CONTENT OUTLINE

- Discuss the need to monitor chronically ill mental patients and those with psychosocial crises in the community.
- Highlight the supportive and preventive roles.

METHOD
Discussion

Competency 20.5

Describe the emerging field of body-mind medicine and its effects on holistic nursing care.

CONTENT OUTLINE

- Define mind modulation.
- Discuss the mind-body connection.
- Describe psychoneuroimmunology as the study of the mind-body connection.

METHOD
Lecture

Competency 20.6

Utilize nursing theory to complete holistic nursing assessments and provide interventions in situations where the client is facing both physical and psychiatric symptoms.

CONTENT OUTLINE

- Identify nursing diagnoses that apply to the emotional care of the patient with physical illness.
- Review the concepts of acceptance, unconditional caring, and holism.
- Describe the usefulness of the theory of modeling and role modeling in holistic care.

METHOD
Discussion
Slide/transparency
Review Table 20-1

Learning Experiences

Theory Application

• Apply the nursing theory of Peplau to the care of the client with emotional needs related to physical illness.

• Discuss the application of cognitive behavioral approaches to care for the person recovering from cardiac surgery.

Individual Activities

• In their journals, have students reflect on their responses to the excerpt titled *Tuesday June 26th*.

• Direct students to imagine living with chronic pain: "In your mind's eye imagine that every time you moved your right upper quadrant, you felt a burning sensation from finger tip to earlobe, from head to buttock. How would this affect *your* day-to-day life? How do you think you would respond?"

Group Activities

• As a class discuss the excerpt titled *A Case Conference*. What other strategies might be applied to Mrs. Bell's case?

• Role Play in two parts: On 3 × 5 cards write the names of several physical illnesses that have strong emotional factors. Have students form dyads and randomly distribute the "diseases."

Part 1: Student A enacts the role of the nurse doing an assessment interview for student B, the client with the disorder.

Part 2: Student A enacts the role of the family member of the ill person while student B acts as the nurse in the interaction.

Clinical Activities

• Review the standard nursing care for oncology patients and identify additional nursing interventions to deal with the emotional care of the client.

• Meet with the enterostomal nurse and discuss the emotional needs of the client who has an ostomy.

Community Applications

• Attend a Reach for Recovery meeting to get a better understanding of the lived experience of emotional aspects to physical illness.

• Contact the state nurses association to find a listing of psychiatric liaison nurses in your locale.

Internet Activities

• A brief overview of the complex interaction of the psychological aspects of neuromuscular disease can be found at this University of California, Davis, site:

http://disability.ucdavis.edu/database/Documents/Psychological_issues/psychaspects.html

• The important role of psychologists as an integral part of the rehabilitation team can be found at this University of California, Davis site:

http://rrtc.ucdavis.edu/pm&r/roleofpsyc.htm

Forgotten Populations: The Homeless and the Incarcerated

Chapter 21

Competencies

Upon completion of this chapter, the learner will be able to:

1. Describe the economic and social factors leading to the number of homeless persons currently in the United States.
2. Assess the basic needs of the homeless population.
3. Describe nursing services and interventions helpful to meeting the needs of the homeless from an individual and a community perspective.
4. Describe the changing and growing population of prisoners in the United States.
5. Identify the major mental health needs and risks for the prison population.
6. Describe the nursing services and interventions helpful in meeting the needs of the incarcerated.

Key Terms

Deinstitutionalization	Incarcerated
Homelessness	NIMBY syndrome

Teaching Methods and Strategies

This chapter focuses on two vulnerable populations: the homeless and the incarcerated. These two groups represent societal concerns as well as concern for the individual's health care needs. The reflective thinking questions in Chapter 21 are designed to help students clarify their own perceptions and understanding of these two groups of clients.

Lesson Plans

Topic: Homeless and Incarcerated Clients

Competency 21.1

Describe the economic and social factors leading to the number of homeless persons currently in the United States.

CONTENT OUTLINE

- Define deinstitutionalization.
- Identify other factors that influence homelessness:
  - Loss of casual nonskilled employment market
  - Closing of short-term single-room housing
  - Availability of crack cocaine and alcohol

METHOD

Lecture
Discussion

Competency 21.2

Assess the basic needs of the homeless population.

CONTENT OUTLINE

- Identify physical needs of the homeless:

Food	Clothing
Shelter	Primary health care

- Identify the psychological/mental health needs of the homeless:

Belonging	Hope
Sense of purpose	Meaning
Identity maintenance	Relationships

METHOD

Discussion

Competency 21.3

Describe nursing services and interventions helpful to meeting the needs of the homeless from an individual and community nursing perspective.

CONTENT OUTLINE

- Identify nursing diagnoses that apply to the mental health and social needs of the homeless:
  - Ineffective individual coping
  - Chemical dependency
  - Social isolation
  - Disturbed self-esteem
  - Hopelessness
  - Powerlessness
  - Disturbed thought processes
  - Disturbed sensory perception
- Identify nursing approaches to working with the homeless, including advocacy and how to negotiate the system:
  - Trusting interpersonal relationships
  - Social support groups
  - Preventive education
  - Emotional support

METHOD

Discussion
Slide/transparency

Competency 21.4

Describe the changing and growing population of prisoners in the United States.

CONTENT OUTLINE

- Describe the changes in the last decade in the number of incarcerated individuals in the United States.
- Describe the changing health needs of the incarcerated population.
- Describe the mental health needs of the incarcerated:

Depression	Substance abuse
Suicide	Psychosis
Personality disorders	

METHOD

Lecture

Competency 21.5

Identify the major mental health needs and risks for the prison population.

CONTENT OUTLINE

- Discuss the need for psychiatric evaluation services for the incarcerated.
- Discuss the need for treatment of depression and psychoses.
- Discuss the need for prevention of suicide among the incarcerated.

METHOD

Discussion

Competency 21.6

Describe the nursing services and interventions helpful to meeting the needs of the incarcerated.

CONTENT OUTLINE

- List relevant nursing diagnoses for the incarcerated client:

Social isolation	Risk for violence
Ineffective individual coping	Risk for suicide
Disturbed self-esteem	Hopelessness
Powerlessness	

- Review the indicators for suicide risk among inmates.
- Discuss the role of advocacy for the psychiatric mental health nurse caring for the incarcerated.

METHOD

Lecture
Discussion
Slide/transparency

Learning Experiences

Theory Application

- Identify nursing strategies that might be useful in caring for a depressed homeless family composed of a man, woman, and 5-year-old child.
- Apply Roy's Adaptation theory to a plan of care for an incarcerated individual who experiences delusions.

Individual Activities

- Have students list three strategies they might use to work with a depressed homeless man to provide care.
- In their journals, have students describe their first reaction to considering caring for a homeless person.

Group Activities

- Discussion: As a class, discuss the societal changes that contributed to the problem of homelessness as described by Jencks.
- Discussion: Are the mental health needs of clients on a forensic psychiatric unit different from those incarcerated in a general county facility? Provide a rationale for your response. If the group identifies the needs as different, provide examples.

Clinical Activities

- Interview a psychiatric nurse who works with the incarcerated.
- Develop a list of health care resources that can be posted in area shelters to assist in providing primary health care services to this group.

Community Applications

- Identify the location of a homeless shelter in the community.
- Assist in a shelter-based health clinic.

Internet Activities

- The Health Resources and Services Administration Bureau of Primary Health Care (of the Department of Health and Human Services) can be reached at:

  http://www.bphc.hrsa.dhhs.gov

- The GAINS Center on Policy Research has publications relating to mental health and the incarcerated individual. Included among the topics are articles addressing the special needs of women with co-occurring disorders in the criminal justice system, jail diversion—creating alternatives for persons with mental illness—and a mental health profile of federally sentenced offenders in Canada:

  http://www.prainc.com/gains/webpub.htm

The Child

Chapter 22

Competencies

Upon completion of this chapter, the learner will be able to:

1. Explain how to assess the emotional, social, and educational needs and problems of children and their families.
2. Describe the common psychiatric disorders of childhood.
3. Apply the nursing process to children with psychiatric disorders through assessment, diagnosis, outcome identification, planning individualized care, and evaluating care based on outcomes.
4. Describe various treatment modalities relevant to the care of children with these disorders.

Key Terms

Asberger's Syndrome	Oppositional Defiant Disorder
Autism	Reactive Depression
Conduct Disorder	Separation Anxiety
Dysthymia	Social Phobia

Teaching Methods and Strategies

Some mental illnesses such as ADHD and Asberger's Syndrome are seen predominantly in children. Others such as depression and anxiety disorders are common also to adulthood.However, the child's experience is, undoubtedly, different from that of an adult's. It is suggested that the criteria for specific disorders be objectively presented and then open a discussion about the human factors of caring for the child in the context of their development and as a part of a family.

The information from previous chapters can be integrated into the discussions, especially information regarding nursing interventions based on specific frameworks. Also, use of vignettes and videos to illustrate the behavioral manifestation of the childhood disorders can be very useful.

Lesson Plans

Topic: The Child

Competency 22.1

Discuss developmental factors which affect the way in which mental illness is experienced by children.

METHOD

Review excerpts from Lenora's Story about childhood Depression by Olive Senior.

Competency 22.2

Explain how to assess the emotional, social, and educational needs and problems of children and their families.

CONTENT OUTLINE

- Emphasize the nurse's therapeutic use of self in the data collection process.
- Identify the importance of collecting data from family members.
- Highlight the importance of identifying behaviors that extend beyond age-appropriateness, are of excessive intensity, or deviate from social or cultural norms.
- Incorporate the use of specific assessment tools and techniques.

METHOD

Lecture

Competency 22.3

Describe the common psychiatric disorders of childhood.

CONTENT OUTLINE

Describe the characteristic behaviors of Attention Deficit Hyperactive Disorder (ADHD).

Discuss the role of genetics and environmental factors in ADHD.

- Describe the characteristic behaviors of childhood depression.
- Describe the characteristic behaviors of Anxiety Disorders in children.
- Describe the characteristic behaviors of Autistic Disorder and Asberger's Syndrome.
- Describe the characteristic behaviors of Disruptive Disorders.
- Discuss the biological and environmental determinants of various Conduct Disorders.

METHOD

Lecture

Competency 22.4

Apply the nursing process to children with psychiatric disorders through assessment, diagnosis, outcome identification, planning individualized care, and evaluating care based on outcomes.

CONTENT OUTLINE

- Identify the elements of a thorough assessment for the child.
- Identify nursing diagnoses applicable to care of the child with a psychiatric disorder:
  - Anxiety
  - Impaired social interaction
  - Isolation
  - Ineffective individual coping
  - Disturbed self-esteem
  - Risk for injury
  - Risk for violence
  - Interrupted family processes

METHOD

Lecture
Slide/transparency
Review the case study/care plan for Jean

Competency 22.5

Describe various treatment modalities relevant to the care of children with these disorders.

CONTENT OUTLINE

- Discuss the use of a therapeutic nurse-client relationship in caring for the child with emotional disorders.
- Discuss the role of play therapy as a treatment modality.
- Discuss individual therapy and family therapy in the treatment of the child.
- Discuss the behavior-modification approach.
- Discuss the role of pharmacological agents for different childhood psychiatric disorders:
  - Antipsychotic medications
  - Antidepressants
  - Anxiolytics
  - Mood stabilizers
  - Stimulants

METHOD

Discussion
Case example

Learning Experiences

Theory Application

• Describe the use of behavior modification in treatment of ADHD.

• Review the major psychopharmacological agents used in treating childhood psychiatric disorders.

Individual Activities

• Encourage students to read the book *Dibs in Search of Self* and reflect on the interactions of the therapist with Dibs.

• Direct the class to review the age-specific symptoms of depression.

Group Activities

• Discussion: What strategies might be used to establish a trusting nurse-client relationship with a child diagnosed with Conduct Disorder?

• Discussion: You are assessing a child of three who witnessed one parent batter a sibling and the other parent. What behaviors are you likely to note or what behaviors might a caregiver report? What strategies might be most useful to assess the child?

Clinical Activities

• Review the DSM-IV-TR diagnostic criteria for the psychiatric disorders of childhood related to anxiety.

• Review and compare the DSM-IV-TR criteria for Attention Deficit Hyperactive Disorder and for Conduct Disorder.

Community Applications

• Visit a community facility where children with psychiatric disorders receive treatment.

• Contact the departments of education and social services to get information about referral resources in the community for children with psychiatric disorders.

• Visit a classroom of children with special needs and one in which a student with special needs is mainstreamed into a regular classroom.

Internet Activities

• Types of childhood mental disorders, warning signs, diagnosis, and treatment information can be found at:
http://www.modmh.state.mo.us/cps/facts/cpschild.html

• Information concerning mental disorders of youth, reading lists, fact sheets, and much more can be found at the National Alliance for the Mentally Ill (NAMI) web site:
http://www.nami.org/youth

• The American Psychiatric Association has a publication for the public about mental disorders of childhood:
http://www.psych.org/public_info/childr~l.cfm

The Adolescent

Chapter 23

Competencies

Upon completion of this chapter, the learner will be able to:

1. Differentiate among various definitions of adolescent mental health.
2. Identify the physical, cognitive, emotional, and social transitions of adolescence.
3. Examine concepts and theories about identity formation and social competence.
4. Reflect on your own sense of personal identity and social competence.
5. Identify major mental health needs and concerns of adolescents.
6. Apply the nursing process to the care of adolescent clients.
7. Integrate nursing theories into planning care for the adolescent in need of mental health services.

Key Terms

Foreclosure
Gender identity
Gender role
Identity achievement
Identity diffusion
Identity Status
Identity formation
Moratorium
Presence
Self-awareness
Self-efficacy
Social competence
Suicidal ideation

Teaching Methods and Strategies

The needs of the adolescent provide the focal point of teaching this content. Due to the many transitions that occur during this phase of life, nursing interventions must remain purposeful yet flexible. Similarly, the approaches used by the educator must be flexible.

Many of the individuals enrolled in a psychiatric nursing class may themselves be in late adolescence. It is helpful for the educator to remain cognizant of this when discussing the mental disorders that may be noted during adolescence. Discussion may be threatening to the student who is struggling with these same normative transitions. Using prepared case studies, videos, and the like can assist in focusing the learning tasks.

Lesson Plans

Topic: The Adolescent

Competency 23.1

Differentiate among various definitions of adolescent mental health.

CONTENT OUTLINE

- Central to healthy adolescence is identity formation and social competence.
- The focus shifts as the adolescent moves through the transitions of each phase:
  Early: Onset of physical changes of puberty
  Middle: Peer pressure to conform
  Late: Commitment to roles and responsibilities

METHOD

Lecture

Competency 23.2

Identify the physical, cognitive, emotional, and social transitions of adolescence.

CONTENT OUTLINE

- Review the physical transitions of adolescence:
  Physical maturation
  Secondary sexual characteristics
  Voice changes
- Review the cognitive transitions of adolescence:
  Impulsivity
  High-risk behaviors
  Experimentation
  Decision making without thought of consequences
- Review the emotional transitions of adolescence:
  Anxiety
  Depression
  Fear
  Confusion
- Review the social transitions of adolescence:
  More time away from family
  Seek out peers
  Experiment with adult-like social behaviors such as work, spending money, leisure time
  Increased conflicts and arguments

METHOD

Lecture

Competency 23.3

Explore concepts and theories about identity formation and social competence.

CONTENT OUTLINE

- Discuss the central concept of developmental theory—identity formation.
- Discuss how adolescents revisit the developmental tasks of earlier stages as they strive for integration.
- Review the statuses of adolescent identity proposed by Marcia:

Foreclosure	Identity diffusion
Moratorium	Identity achievement

- Describe the social learning theory concepts of social competence, self-efficacy, and self-awareness.

METHOD

Lecture
Review Table 23-1

Competency 23.4

Reflect on your own sense of personal identity and social competence.

CONTENT OUTLINE

- Encourage students to identify where they are in their own journey of identity formation and social formation.
- Focus on the excerpts in this chapter to highlight different perspectives about identity and competence.

METHOD

Discussion
Case example

Competency 23.5

Identify major mental health needs and concerns of adolescents.

CONTENT OUTLINE

- Identify mental health needs reflective of adolescent transitions:

Anxiety	Body image distortion
Social isolation	Alteration in relationships

- Identify mental health disorders and concerns experienced by adolescents:

Conduct Disorder	Suicide risk
Anorexia Nervosa	Gender Identity Disorder
Depression	

- Discuss adolescent needs related to social factors such as poverty, lack of health role models, and violence.

METHOD

Lecture

Competency 23.6

Apply the nursing process to the care of adolescent clients.

CONTENT OUTLINE

- Using the case study of Ms. Ivanhoe, identify each phase of the nursing process.
- Identify the nursing diagnoses most applicable to the care of the adolescent with depression, Conduct Disorder, and Anorexia Nervosa.

METHOD

Discussion
Slide/transparency
Case example

Competency 23.7

Integrate nursing theories into planning care for the adolescent in need of mental health services.

CONTENT OUTLINE

- Review the 12 behaviors for providing humanistic nursing care.
- Apply the framework of Newman (expanding human consciousness) to care of the adolescent.

METHOD

Discussion
Case example

Learning Experiences

Theory Application

- Apply developmental theory to the case of Ms. Ivanhoe.
- Review suicide assessment information and apply it specifically to the adolescent.

Individual Activities

- In their journals, have students reflect on their own adolescent transitions.
- Encourage students to reflect on their responses to reading the excerpts from *When Rabbit Howls.*

Group Activities

- Discussion: What strategies can be suggested to parents of adolescents to ease this transition period?
- Discussion: What nursing strategies would you use in working with Truddi?

Clinical Activities

- Engage in a group discussion with several adolescents about what their biggest concerns are related to mental illness.

• Interview the staff on an eating disorders unit to get their perspective and responses to dealing with the adolescent diagnosed with anorexia.

Community Applications

• Identify the resources in the community to assist adolescents with potential psychiatric problems.

• Present an awareness seminar at a local high school about suicide prevention.

Internet Activities

• Health issues for young people with a quiz and description of mental illness concerns can be accessed via:

http://www.public.health.wa.gov.au/hp5673.htm

• The web page with resources and publications of the American Academy for Child and Adolescent Psychiatry:

http://www.aacap.org

• Information books about adolescents and suicide, such as Schneidman's *For Whom the Bell Tolls: The Epidemiology of Adolescent Suicide* can be found on the APA web site at:

http://www.apa.org/books

NOTES

The Elderly

Chapter 24

Competencies

Upon completion of this chapter, the learner will be able to:

1. Recognize the interconnected role that physical and family support systems play in the mental health of older adults.
2. Identify pathological processes that are responsible for the disorders of cognition and affect most commonly seen in the older adult.
3. Analyze how ageist stereotypes and socioeconomic factors affect the occurrence of mental illness in the elderly.
4. Describe the most common physiological causes (risk factors) of delirium and acute confusion states in the elderly.
5. Describe the genetic basis and pharmacological processes of Alzheimer's.
6. Envision and illustrate ways in which severe memory loss poses a challenge to self-concept and human dignity.
7. Propose nursing interventions for demented elders and their caregivers that are derived from a caring framework.
8. Identify environmental and physiological risk factors for depression in the elderly.
9. Explain the basis for treatment modalities of depression in older adults.

Key Terms

Aphasia	Confusion
Catastrophic reaction	Delirium
Cognition	Dementia
Confabulation	Mutuality

Teaching Methods and Strategies

With the ever-growing cohort of elderly, it is imperative that nursing education incorporate more experiences in providing care to the elderly experiencing psychiatric illness. Few students have experienced living within multigenerational homes with elders diagnosed with psychiatric problems. Nursing homes and day care of the elderly are also areas where such elder clients receive care. The educator can draw upon these resources to more vividly illustrate the nursing concerns for the elderly and their caregivers.

Lesson Plans

Topic: The Elderly

Competency 24.1

Recognize the interconnected role that physical health and family support systems play in the mental health of older adults.

CONTENT OUTLINE

- Identify factors that place the older individual at risk for mental health problems:
  - Physical frailty
  - Chronic illnesses
  - Threats to identity and esteem
  - Frequent losses
  - Inadequate social support
  - Low socioeconomic position
- Reflect on the increased vulnerability of the aging brain to internal and external environmental factors.

METHOD

Lecture
Discussion

Competency 24.2

Identify pathological processes that are responsible for the disorders of cognition and affect most commonly seen in the older adult.

CONTENT OUTLINE

- Identify the pathological processes and characteristic behaviors associated with delirium:
  - Pathology (reversible)
    - General medical conditions
    - Drug toxicity
    - Infection
    - Fluid and electrolyte imbalance, dehydration
    - Hepatic or renal disease
    - Hypoxia
    - Metabolic disorders
    - Nutritional deficiencies

Behaviors (reversible)
- Clouding of consciousness
- Difficulty maintaining attention
- Illusions or hallucinations
- Disorganized thinking
- Unfocused speech
- Disoriented to time and place
- Strong emotional reactions
- Memory impairment

- Identify the pathological processes and characteristic behaviors associated with depression in the elderly:

  Pathology
  - Physical illness
  - Neurotransmitter deficit and reduced sensitivity of receptors
  - Chronically elevated cortisol levels related to dysregulation of the hypothalamus-pituitary-adrenal feedback mechanism
  - Unfulfilled desires/accomplishments
  - Losses
  - Lack of social supports
  - Poverty
  - Isolation
  - Loss of role status
  - Financial strain

  Behaviors (as with depression)
  - Emotional, physical, social, cognitive
  - Risk for suicide
  - Subtypes of depression:
    Major clinical depression
    Dysthymic disorder
    Adjustment disorder with depressed mood
    Grief and bereavement

- Identify the pathological processes and characteristic behaviors associated with different types of dementia:

  Pathology
  - Infections
  - Degenerative neurological disorders
  - Vascular disorders
  - Structural disorders of brain tissue

  Behaviors (gradual onset)
  - Multiple cognitive deficits
  - Memory impairment
  - Aphasia
  - Apraxia
  - Agnosia
  - Disturbance of executive functioning
  - Delayed response time
  - Paranoia
  - Catastrophic reactions
  - Perceptual alterations
  - Wandering
  - Disinhibition

  Types
  - Primary dementia, Alzheimer's type
  - Vascular dementia
  - Other dementia

METHOD

Lecture
Discussion
Slide/transparency

Competency 24.3

Analyze how ageist stereotypes and socioeconomic factors affect the occurrence of mental illness in the elderly.

CONTENT OUTLINE

- Discuss socioeconomic factors that influence the mental health of the elderly individual.
- Discuss ageist perspectives about aging and youth.

METHOD

Discussion

Competency 24.4

Describe the most common physiological causes (risk factors) of delirium and acute confusion states in the elderly.

CONTENT OUTLINE

- List the related pathologies:
  Brain tumors
  Dehydration
  Drug toxicity
  Electrolyte imbalances
  Hepatic and renal problems
  Hypoxia (secondary to respiratory and circulatory disorders)
  Hyper- or hypothermia
- Discuss the significance of polypharmacy in the elderly client.

METHOD

Lecture

Competency 24.5

Describe the genetic basis and pathological processes of Alzheimer's.

CONTENT OUTLINE

- Identify chromosomal abnormalities associated with:
  Early onset
  Late onset.
- Describe the inflammatory and structural changes associated with Alzheimer's:
  Beta-amyloid plaque and APOE
  Abnormal tau and neurofibrillary tangles.

- Describe the purpose and basis for pharmacological treatment of Alzheimer's as it relates to the pathophysiology:
  - Cholinergics
  - Antiinflammatories and free-radical scavengers
  - Folate, Vitamins B6 and B12

METHOD

Lecture
Discussion

Competency 24.6

Envision and illustrate ways in which severe memory loss poses a challenge to self-concept and human dignity.

CONTENT OUTLINE

- Discuss the frustration associated with inability to communicate thoughts.
- Discuss the impact on sense of self, meaning, and esteem related to the disorders of cognition.

METHOD

Lecture
Discussion

Competency 24.7

Propose nursing interventions for demented elders and their caregivers that are derived from a caring framework.

CONTENT OUTLINE

- Identify the nursing diagnoses associated with collaborative physiological dysfunctions:
  - Deficient fluid volume
  - Imbalanced nutrition
  - Risk for infection
  - Ineffective tissue perfusion
- Identify nursing diagnoses associated with brain dysfunctions:
  - Disturbed sensory perception
  - Impaired verbal communication
  - Disturbed thought processes
  - Disturbed sleep pattern
- Identify nursing diagnoses associated with threats to dignity and safety:
  - Powerlessness
  - Self-care deficit
  - Disturbed personal identity
  - Fear
  - Risk for injury
  - Anxiety

METHOD

Lecture
Discussion
Slide/transparency
Review Table 24-1

Competency 24.8

Identify environmental and physiological risk factors for depression in the elderly.

CONTENT OUTLINE

- Identify environmental factors:
  - Isolation
  - Low socioeconomic status
  - Institutionalization
  - Loss of status
  - Death of a loved one
- Identify physiological risk factors:
  - Lowered neurotransmitter levels
  - Hypoxia
  - Dysregulation of hypothalamic-pituitary-adrenal feedback loop
  - Depressogenic medications
- Discuss the link between illness and depression:
  - Alzheimer's
  - Pain
  - Chronic and acute illness

METHOD

Lecture

Competency 24.9

Explain the basis for treatment modalities of depression in older adults.

CONTENT OUTLINE

- Discuss the need for a multifaceted approach to care.
- Discuss the challenge of pharmacological treatment in the elderly.

METHOD

Lecture
Discussion

Learning Experiences

Theory Application

- Review the DSM-IV-TR diagnostic criteria for disorders of cognition.
- Discuss new pharmacological interventions for disorders of cognition.

Individual Activities

- Direct students to prepare a list of questions to use to assess categories of cognitive functioning in an elderly client.
- In their journals, ask students to react to the excerpt titled *A Crabbit Old Woman.*

Group Activities

- Small Group Discussion: Divide the class into groups of 5–8 and discuss responses to the literary excerpts in the chapter.
- Panel: Divide the students into three groups. Instruct them to develop three questions to ask the caregiver of

an elderly client with a designated type of psychiatric illness (depression, Alzheimer's, vascular dementia).

• Invite several caregivers of elderly clients with mental illnesses to present their experiences and respond to student questions.

Clinical Activities

• Experience the process of interviewing an elderly person diagnosed with dementia.

• Using the geriatric depression scale, interview an elderly client.

Community Applications

• Identify agencies in the community that provide respite care for caregivers of the mentally ill elderly client.

• Contact the county agency responsible for programs for the aged and request resource lists to distribute.

Internet Activities

• Many resources related to depression in the elderly can be found via psycom.net. It includes an overview of the problem of depression among the elderly; information about diagnosis, treatment, and medications; a self-administered depression scale; and tips about suicide prevention:

http://www.psycom.net/depression.central.elderly.html

• Listings of organizations and resources on aging and mental health are part of the APA division dedicated to the psychology of adult development and aging:

http://aging.ufl.edu/apadiv20/clingd5.htm

• Visit the website of the Rosalyn Carter Institue for Human Development which is dedicated to building public awareness of caregiving needs:

http://rci.gsw.edu

Survivors of Violence or Abuse

Chapter 25

Competencies

Upon completion of this chapter, the learner will be able to:

1. Identify the major theories that explain why interpersonal violence occurs.
2. Identify factors that may contribute to interpersonal violence.
3. Define general types of family violence: physical, psychological, financial, and sexual abuse and neglect.
4. Identify the typical indicators of abuse and neglect observed in interpersonal relationships and the characteristics of the abusers.
5. Describe the nurse's legal responsibility in regards to child and elder abuse mandatory reporting laws and clients who have been sexually assaulted.
6. Describe the cycle of domestic violence.
7. Utilize crisis intervention techniques in interviewing in cases of family violence and sexual assault.
8. Utilize community resources that are available to prevent abuse and to assist survivors and perpetrators in abusive situations.
9. Apply the nursing process to clients who are abused and neglected by:
   - Performing nursing assessments for abuse and neglect
   - Analyzing data in terms of nursing and crisis theories
   - Formulating individual nursing diagnoses
   - Deriving a plan of care
   - Evaluating care based on resolution of the abuse and neglect

Key Terms

Acquaintance (date) rape
Aggravated criminal sexual assault
Child abuse
Child molestation
Child pornography
Criminal sexual assault
Domestic violence
Financial abuse
Forcible rape
Gang rape
Incest
Mental injury
Negligent treatment
Passive physical abuse (negligence)
Physical abuse
Physical injury
Psychological abuse
Rape
Sexual abuse—child
Sexual abuse—elder
Sexual battery
Sexual exploitation
Sexually explicit conduct
Spousal rape
Statutory rape
Stranger rape
Violation of rights

Teaching Methods and Strategies

This chapter has many informative boxes of information that can facilitate presenting the information. The educator can refer directly to the text or develop transparencies from the boxed information. The thematic link for the information in Chapter 25 is violence. By first presenting the information about theories of violence and the cycle of violence, the specific information about abuse, rape, and domestic violence can be compared and contrasted.

Lesson Plans

Topic: Violence and Abuse

Competency 25.1

Identify the major theories that explain why interpersonal violence occurs.

CONTENT OUTLINE

- Discuss violence as influenced by a complex interaction of personal, psychological, social, and environmental factors.
- Biological theory emphasizes violence as innate and instinctual; due to hormonal imbalances.
- Analytical framework points to personality traits that need to discharge hostility and aggression due to ego weakness.
- Social learning theory hypothesizes that aggressive behavior is part of the socialization process, a learned response through modeling, observing, and direct experience.

METHOD

Lecture
Slide/transparency

Competency 25.2

Identify factors that may contribute to interpersonal violence.

CONTENT OUTLINE

- Discuss societal influences that contribute to interpersonal violence.
- Discuss the potential role of severe physical disciplining, psychological abuse, and neglect in development of interpersonal violence.

METHOD

Discussion

Competency 25.3

Define general types of family violence: physical, psychological, financial, and sexual abuse and neglect.

CONTENT OUTLINE

- Define terms associated with child abuse and neglect:

Child abuse	Sexually explicit conduct
Negligent treatment	Child molestation
Physical injury	Sexual exploitation
Mental injury	Incest
Sexual abuse	

- Describe abuse as related to the complex interaction of variables including social, financial, and relationship variables.

METHOD

Discussion

Review the list of definitions adopted from the Victims of Child Abuse Act of 1990

Competency 25.4

Identify the typical indicators of abuse and neglect observed in interpersonal relationships and the characteristics of the abusers.

CONTENT OUTLINE

- Review characteristics of child abuse and neglect:
  - *Physical:* Bruises, bite marks, burns, fractures, lacerations, shaken-baby syndrome, chunks of hair missing
  - *Neglect*: Malnourished, poor skin care, tired, lethargic, lack of needed medical care, unsupervised for extended periods
  - *Behavior:* Late or absent from school, poor school performance, acts unpleasant or demanding, oppositional, wary of adults, anxious to please, breaks and damages things, begs or steals food, uses alcohol/drugs, engages in vandalism, sexual misconduct, wears clothes to conceal, seems frightened of parents, reports injury by parent
- Review the characteristic symptoms of sexual abuse in children:
  - *Physical:* Itching, bruising, bleeding, edema, pain in external genitalia, vagina, anal area, cervix; pain or injury to mouth; vaginal or penile discharge; bladder infections; STD
  - *Verbal:* Reports sexual activity to friend, teacher, nurse; physical complaints; indirect statements about abuse or sexual assault
  - *Behavioral:* Torn, stained, bloody undergarments; regression; temper tantrums; acting out behavior with toys, animals, other people; sexual promiscuity; preoccupation with sexual organs; altered sleep patterns; feelings of fear, anger, guilt, shame, confusion; delinquency, acting out; phobias, avoidant behaviors, depression
- Review characteristics of elder abuse and neglect:
  - *Physical:* Bruises in various stages of healing or under clothing or in genital areas; unexplained fractures, internal injuries, or bleeding; dehydration or malnourishment without illness-related cause; fecal/urine smell; lack of heat or air conditioing; decubiti; constantly soiled clothing or bed.
  - *Psychological:* Sleep disturbances; Irritable and anxious; frequent crying; extreme withdrawal; loss of interest in usual activities; confusion, disorientation, or unusual behaviors such as rocking or sucking; hesitation to talk openly or nonresponsiveness; anger; suicidal talk.
  - *Financial*: Sudden changes in bank account or banking practices; forged elder's signature; abrupt changes in a will.
  - *Caregiver behaviors:* Treats the elderly person like an infant; refuses to spend money on the care of elder which may result in numerous unpaid bills; refuses to allow visitors to see elder alone; blames the elder; history of abusive behavior; gives conflicting accounts of incidents.

METHOD

Lecture

Slide/transparency

Review boxed information

Competency 25.5

Describe the nurse's legal responsibility in regards to child and elder abuse mandatory reporting laws and clients who have been sexually assaulted.

CONTENT OUTLINE

- Discuss mandatory reporting laws related to abuse.
- Discuss procedures required to report abuse.

METHOD

Discussion

Competency 25.6

Describe the cycle of domestic violence.

CONTENT OUTLINE

- Identify the goal of domestic violence as power and control.
- Describe the elements of domestic violence:

Intimidation	Sexual abuse
Isolation	Threats
Emotional abuse	Using children
Economic abuse	Using male privilege

- Review the characteristics of battered women:
  - Low self-esteem
  - Believe myths about battering relationships
  - Subscribe to female sex role stereotype

Accept responsibility for batterer's actions
Feel guilty and ashamed
Deny anger and terror they feel
Have severe stress reactions/psychosomatic complaints, chronic pain
Soft tissue injuries
Self-destructive behaviors
Sleep disturbances
View self as victim

- Review the characteristics of men who batter:
  Low self-esteem
  Believe myths about battering relationships
  Believe stereotype of male privilege
  Blame others for actions
  Pathologically jealous
  Self-destructive behaviors (drugs, alcohol)
  Sex is act of aggression to enhance self-esteem
  Seek second chance; believe battering should not have negative consequences
  Charming, gregarious, or gentle to nonfamily

METHOD

Lecture
Slide/transparency
Video

Competency 25.7

Utilize crisis intervention techniques in interviewing in cases of family violence and sexual assault.

CONTENT OUTLINE

- Review crisis interventions.
- Apply crisis interventions to caring for the victim of violence.

METHOD

Lecture
Case example

Competency 25.8

Utilize community resources that are available to prevent abuse and to assist survivors and perpetrators in abusive situations.

CONTENT OUTLINE

- Identify the role of the community nurse in case finding.
- Describe alternative living arrangements used for victims of violence.
- Discuss the limitations of community resources for dealing with the survivors.

METHOD

Lecture

Competency 25.9

Apply the nursing process to clients who are abused and neglected by:

- Performing nursing assessments for abuse and neglect
- Analyzing data in terms of nursing and crisis theories
- Formulating individual nursing diagnoses
- Deriving a plan of care
- Evaluating care based on resolution of the abuse and neglect

CONTENT OUTLINE

- Review the NANDA diagnoses applicable to caring for the abused or neglected client related to:

Choosing	Perceiving
Feeling	Relating
Knowing	Valuing

- Review the NANDA defining characteristics applicable to the aforementioned nursing diagnoses.
- Discuss the nursing interventions for caring for the client who experiences violence.

METHOD

Discussion
Slide/transparency
Case example
Review boxed information

Learning Experiences

Theory Application

- Review, in depth, the "Wheel of Power and Control" presented in Figure 25-1.
- Review the stages of prevention and apply them to all forms of violence discussed in this chapter.

Individual Activities

- Have students reflect on their feelings about the excerpt titled "Prized Possessions" in their journals.
- Review what you would do if a friend confided in you that she had been sexually assaulted.

Group Activities

- Discussion: Discuss the myths about rape and about domestic violence presented in Tables 25-1 and 25-2.
- Discussion: Using the case study, discuss the possible responses of the nursing staff while attending to Elizabeth.

Clinical Activities

- Review the JCAHO-approved protocol for examining and treating victims of violence and assault in the facility.

• Review the documentation procedure for interpersonal violence and sexual abuse situations.

Community Applications

• Identify rape crisis resources in your community.

• Working with the guidance counselor, facilitate a group discussion at a community junior high school about the myths associated with violence and sexual abuse and facts.

Internet Activities

• This web site offers information about sexual abuse, signs and symptoms, overt and covert abuse (including verbal, boundary violation, and emotional abuse), and dealing with the aftereffects:

http://www.golden.net/~soul/sexab.html

• Numerous websites are available by typing in "rape and sexual assault resources" at:

http://www.msn.com

• "Stop Prisoner Rape" combats the rape of male and female prisoners and provides assistance to survivors of prison rape:

http://www.spr.org

Unit 4

Nursing Interventions and Treatment Modalities

The chapters in Unit 4 provide the information needed to understand the treatment modalities and approaches that are generally used for care of the client in psychiatric mental health settings. Chapter 26 presents the foundational information on the use of medications. The essentials of psychopharmacology and the specifics of medications useful in the treatment of certain disorders are covered in this chapter.

Perspectives of different therapies available to people with mental illness appear in Chapters 27 through 29. These chapters include individual therapies (Chapter 27), family therapies (Chapter 28), and group therapies (Chapter 29). The nurse's role in supporting each approach, as well as nursing theoretical perspectives, are included within each chapter.

Chapter 30 shifts the focus to aggregate mental health needs. The role of the nurse in community mental health and the services needed for comprehensive mental health centers are delineated. In addition, the last chapter, Chapter 31, presents an overview of some of the complementary approaches to care.

NOTES

Pharmacology in Psychiatric Care

Chapter 26

Competencies

Note: the competencies listed below, derived from the competencies that appear at the beginning of the chapter, include additional detail to assist the educator in presenting the wealth of information in this chapter.

Upon completion of this chapter, the learner will be able to:

1. Describe the indications, actions, interactions, side effects, and adverse effects of antipsychotic medications.
2. Describe the indications, actions, interactions, side effects, and adverse effects of antidepressant medications.
3. Describe the indications, actions, interactions, side effects, and adverse effects of mood-stabilizing medications.
4. Describe the indications, actions, interactions, side effects, and adverse effects of the anxiolytic and hypnotic medications.
5. Describe the indications, actions, interactions, side effects, and adverse effects of stimulant medications.
6. Describe the indications, actions, interactions, side effects, and adverse effects of drugs used to treat chemical dependency.

Key Terms

- Akathisia
- Antipsychotic drugs
- Blood-brain barrier
- Dystonia
- Half-life
- Neuroleptic malignant syndrome
- Oculogyric crisis
- Serotonergic syndrome
- Tardive dyskinesia
- Therapeutic window

Teaching Methods and Strategies

The information in this chapter is of paramount importance in providing effective and safe nursing care. It is advisable to spend a good amount of time on this content. The indications, actions, interactions, side effects, and adverse effects of each of the major groupings of psychotropic medications are presented. In Tables 26-1, 26-2, and 26-3 a wealth of information has been summarized. It is suggested that the educator use these tables to emphasize the importance of this information and use the summary tables to reinforce the information.

Lesson Plans

Topic: Pharmacology

Competency 26.1

Describe the indications, actions, interactions, side effects, and adverse effects of antipsychotic medications

CONTENT OUTLINE

- Describe indications for antipsychotic medications administered to control "positive" symptoms of psychosis:
  - Hallucinations
  - Delusions
  - Disorganized thought processes
  - Paranoia
- Describe the actions of antipsychotic medications:
  - Act by blocking dopamine D_2 receptors (some also block D_1 and D_4 receptors)
  - Bind to dopamine receptors in the brain
  - Effectiveness dependent on route and form:
    - IM within 15–30 minutes
    - oral within 1 to 4 hours
- Describe potential drug interactions of antipsychotic medications:
  - Drugs that influence rate of hepatic detoxification
  - Cimetidine (Tagamet) reduces antipsychotic effectiveness
  - Anticonvulsants lower plasma concentrations of antipsychotics
  - Tricyclic antidepressants effects increase when used with antipsychotics
  - Some cardiac drugs may interact with antipsychotics, worsening psychosis
- Describe the side effects of antipsychotic medications:
  - Anticholinergic effects:
    - Constipation
    - Dry mouth
    - Blurred vision
    - Postural hypotension
    - Urinary hesitancy/retention
    - Weight gain
    - Sedation

- Describe the adverse effects of antipsychotic medications:
  - Movement disorders
    - Akathisia
    - Dystonia
    - Tardive dyskinesia
    - Neuroleptic Malignant Syndrome

METHOD

Lecture
Slide/transparency
Review Table 26-1

Competency 26.2

Describe the indications, actions, interactions, side effects, and adverse effects of antidepressant medications.

CONTENT OUTLINE

- Describe indications for antidepressant medications:
  - Relieve symptoms of depression
- Describe the actions of the three classic categories of antidepressant medications (action depends on category of antidepressant):
  - Tricyclics affect reabsorption of neurotransmitters
  - Selective serotonin reuptake inhibitor (SSRI) blocks reabsorption of serotonin
  - Monoamine oxidase inhibitors (MAOI) block the enzyme monoamine oxidase needed to metabolize norepinephrine, serotonin, and dopamine
- Identify most recent antidepressant drugs designed to have fewer side-effects and a more rapid onset of action:
  - Serotonin noradrenergic reuptake inhibitors (SNaRIs)
  - Selective noradrenaline reuptake inhibitors (NaRIs)
  - Noradrenergic and specific serotonergic antidepressants (NaSSAs)
- Describe potential drug interactions of antidepressant medications:
  - *Tricyclics:* Anticholinergic drugs, antipsychotics, antihistamines, anesthesia, narcotic pain relievers, SSRIs, and MAOIs
  - *SSRIs:* Rare, with MAOI can cause serotonergic syndrome
  - *MAOIs:* Antidepressants, narcotic analgesics, preparations containing sympathomimetic drugs (epinephrine, norepinephrine, phenylephrine, isoproterenol, methoxymine), tyramine-containing foods
- Describe the side effects of antidepressant medications:
  - *Tricyclics:* Anticholinergic effects, antihistiminic effects, alpha-adrenergic effects, antidopaminergic effects
  - *SSRIs:* Headache, anxiety, GI disturbance, decreased libido
  - *MAOIs:* Decreased heart rate, hypotension, anticholinergic symptoms, CNS symptoms, sexual dysfunction, weight gain, peripheral neuropathy
- Describe the adverse effects of antidepressant medications:
  - *Tricyclics:* Overdose
  - *SSRIs:* Generally free of adverse effects
  - *MAOIs:* Syncope, bone marrow suppression

METHOD

Lecture
Slide/transparency
Review Table 26-2

Competency 26.3

Describe the indications, actions, interactions, side effects, and adverse effects of mood-stabilizing medications.

CONTENT OUTLINE

- Describe indications for mood-stabilizing medications for control of mania.
- Describe the actions of mood-stabilizing medications:
  - Actual mechanism of action unknown
  - Lithium—as a metallic salt—may affect the way neurotransmitters react
- Describe potential drug interactions of mood-stabilizing medications:
  - Anything that influences sodium levels influences lithium
  - Anything that affects renal functioning influences effectiveness of lithium
  - Anything that influences liver functioning might affect carbamazepine treatment
- Describe the side effects of mood-stabilizing medications:
  - Lithium: Toxicity, arrhythmias
  - Carbamazepine: Dizziness, drowsiness, agranulocytosis
  - Divalproex: Few, rare
- Describe the adverse effects of mood-stabilizing medications:
  - Lithium: Fatal cardiac arrhythmias

METHOD

Lecture
Slide/transparency
Review boxed information: Assessing for Lithium Toxicity

Competency 26.4

Describe the indications, actions, interactions, side effects, and adverse effects of the anxiolytic and hypnotic medications.

CONTENT OUTLINE

- Describe indications for anxiolytic and hypnotic medications:
  For treatment of anxiety disorders and sleep disorders
- Describe the actions of anxiolytic and hypnotic medications:
  Block GABA-nergic CNS pathways to produce sedation, decrease subjective anxiety
- Describe potential drug interactions of anxiolytic and hypnotic medications:
  Alcohol causes additive effect
- Describe the side effects of anxiolytic and hypnotic medications:
  Sedation
- Describe the adverse effects of anxiolytic and hypnotic medications:
  Intentional overdose
  Abuse, physical dependence

METHOD

Lecture
Slide/transparency
Review Table 26-3

Competency 26.5

Describe the indications, actions, interactions, side effects, and adverse effects of stimulant medications.

CONTENT OUTLINE

- Describe indications for stimulant medications:
  Management of Attention Deficit Hyperactive Disorder and management of Narcolepsy
- Describe the actions of stimulant medications.
- Describe potential drug interactions of stimulant medications.
- Describe the side effects of stimulant medications.
- Describe the adverse effects of stimulant medications.

METHOD

Lecture
Discussion

Competency 26.6

Describe the indications, actions, interactions, side effects, and adverse effects of drugs used to treat chemical dependency.

CONTENT OUTLINE

- Describe indications for drugs used to treat chemical dependency:
  Useful for detoxification, overdose, withdrawal
  Depends on medication:
  - *Methadone:* Acute and long-term maintenance of opioid dependence, decrease intensity of withdrawal symptoms
  - *Disulfiram:* For alcohol abstinence
  - *Opioid receptor antagonists* (naloxone nalmefene, naltrexone): For narcotic overdose
  - *Nicotine replacement and long-acting Bupripion:* For smoking addiction withdrawal
- Describe the actions of drugs used to treat chemical dependency:
  Methadone: Binds with opioid receptor sites
  Disulfiram: Inhibits dehydrogenase
  Opioid receptor antagonists: Block effects of opioids
  Nicotine: Attaches to nicotinic receptors so person does not feel severe effects of withdrawal from smoking
- Describe potential drug interactions of drugs used to treat chemical dependency.
- Describe the side effects of drugs used to treat chemical dependency:
  Withdrawal symptoms
- Describe the adverse effects of drugs used to treat chemical dependency.

METHOD

Lecture

Learning Experiences

Theory Application

- Review the basics of pharmacokinetics.
- Review the neurotransmitter responses of psychopharmacological therapies.

Individual Activities

- Direct students to review psychopharmacological agents in a general pharmacology text.
- Have students review the information in Tables 26-1 through 26-3.

Group Activities

- Debate: The pros and cons of methadone treatment

Divide the group in half and assign one half to investigate the pro position and the other half to investigate the con position. The following class, redivide the groups into smaller teams (three pro and three con representatives in each group) and have them debate each other. Use the debate format with each side exchanging information:

3 minutes to present position, 3 minutes for rebuttal, 2 minutes for counter rebuttal, and 1 minute for summary. Then have students freely discuss the experience.

• Seminar: Assign students to present about each category of psychopharmacologic agents from the perspective of nursing administration, monitoring, and general management. Include important aspects for "med-ed" for clients.

Clinical Activities

• Create a list of the major drugs in each category of psychopharmacologic agents that are used in the specific clinical agency.

• Review the clinical implications of psychopharmacological agents for pregnant and lactating clients.

Internet Activities

• Mental Health Net offers a listing titled "Professional Resources on Psychopharmacology & Drugs." The student can look up drugs by name, access a general database, related newsgroups, journals, and publications:

http://www.mentalhelp.net/guide/pro22.htm

• The American Psychological Association Division on Psychopharmacology and Substance Abuse can be reached via:

http://www.apa.org/divisions/div28

Individual Psychotherapy

Chapter 27

Competencies

Upon completion of this chapter, the learner will be able to:

1. Define psychotherapy.
2. Describe various approaches to therapy including:
   - Psychoanalysis
   - Psychodynamic therapy
   - Interpersonal therapy
   - Cognitive-behavioral therapy
   - Client-centered therapy
3. Suggest ways that psychotherapeutic approaches are used in nursing practice.
4. Relate major psychotherapeutic approaches to nursing theory.
5. Describe the research base of psychotherapeutic interventions.

Key Terms

Catharsis	Interpersonal therapy
Clarification	Interpretation
Client-centered therapy	Manipulation
Cognitive-behavioral therapy	Psychoanalysis
Confrontation	Psychodynamic therapy
Experience-oriented therapy	Psychotherapy
Insight-oriented therapy	Repression
	Suggestion
	Task-oriented therapy

Teaching Methods and Strategies

There are multiple approaches available for individual therapy. This chapter provides a sampling of some of the therapies. The content is brief and more of a sampling than an in-depth explanation of therapy.

Because the students are preparing to be generalist nurses, it is suggested that the educator emphasize the need for understanding the approaches to better provide care: It may be useful to remind the students that they are providing therapy. Psychotherapy is part of the role of the advanced practice psychiatric nurse. Although the distinction between counseling and psychotherapy may seem vague, emphasize to the students that psychotherapy is more intense and requires additional education and experience. Place the emphasis on providing care using the nursing theoretical frameworks that support the various therapies.

Lesson Plans

Topic: Individual Psychotherapy

Competency 27.1

Define psychotherapy.

CONTENT OUTLINE

- Define psychotherapy as the use of techniques to help a person overcome mental distress and to reach their optimal level of health.
- Describe some reasons nurses need to understand psychotherapy:
  - Its effectiveness is supported by data
  - Techniques may parallel/be similar to nursing
  - It has potential relevance to all settings
  - To assist client in making informed decisions
- Various professionals can provide psychotherapy:
  - Psychiatrist
  - Psychologist
  - Psychiatric social worker
  - Advanced practice psychiatric nurse

METHOD

Lecture

Review boxed information: Differing Kinds of Therapies

Competency 27.2

Describe various approaches to therapy.

CONTENT OUTLINE

- Describe psychoanalysis:
  - Based on Freudian theoretical framework
  - Goal of treatment is to demonstrate to client how unconscious factors affect current relationships and behavior patterns
  - Treatment traces patterns back to origins in infancy and childhood
  - The process of repression keeps painful memories and experiences out of consciousness

Assume the client actively resists coming to an understanding of repressed, unconscious thoughts

Techniques used include:

- Suggestion
- Catharsis
- Manipulation
- Confrontation
- Clarification
- Interpretation

• Describe psychodynamic therapy:

Evolved from psychoanalytic principles and interpretations

Uses process that focuses on selected therapeutic issues, so it is brief by comparison to analysis

Assumptions:

- Client desires therapy and will work as hard as possible with the therapist
- Client has basic abilities of cognition and insight

• Describe interpersonal therapy:

Insight based on the recognition that psychological distress occurs in conjunction with disturbed human relationships

Uses the theories of Sullivan

Related nursing theories of Peplau

Relationship with therapist is a positive therapeutic relationship

Client can transfer positive relationship experience outside of therapy session

• Describe cognitive-behavioral therapy:

Concerned with how client thinks about himself

Goals are to:

- Provide cost-effective care for a wide range of problems
- Alter client's interpretations of self by directly changing behavior, environment, cognition
- Increase client's coping skills
- Increase likelihood that gains made during therapy will be maintained
- Be task-oriented; homework assignments given
- Focus on making practical changes
- Frequently use this approach for treating depression

• Describe client-centered therapy:

Experience oriented

Client is agent of change with therapist as facilitator

Therapy provides new ways of being and experiencing

Client's inner resources are brought to light

Therapist is open, nonjudgmental, empathic, respectful of client autonomy, supportive

METHOD

Lecture

Discussion

Competency 27.3

Suggest ways that psychotherapeutic approaches are used in nursing practice.

CONTENT OUTLINE

- Describe usefulness of cognitive techniques to help client examine thought patterns.
- Discuss the fundamentals of client-centered interactions as the basis for therapy and nurse-client relationship.

METHOD

Discussion

Competency 27.4

Relate major psychotherapeutic approaches to nursing theory.

CONTENT OUTLINE

- Relate Peplau's nursing theory to psychodynamic therapy approaches.
- Describe how cognitive-behavioral therapy is consistent with Roy's theory of adaptation.
- Describe the similarities between experience-oriented therapy and the nursing concepts of human care and caring found in the theories of Leininger, Watson, and Erickson.

METHOD

Discussion

Competency 27.5

Describe the research base of psychotherapeutic interventions.

CONTENT OUTLINE

- Describe indications for psychodynamic therapy.
- Describe outcomes of studies of the effectiveness of cognitive and cognitive-behavioral therapy.
- Describe lack of outcome studies for experience-oriented and client-centered therapies.

METHOD

Lecture

Learning Experiences

Theory Application

• Review the theoretical frameworks of the interpersonal psychiatric approach.

• Review the cognitive-behavioral therapy concepts of cognitive distortions and irrational beliefs.

Individual Activities

• After reviewing the approaches to individual therapy, have students discuss which one they might find most interesting to know more about and explain why.

• Select a therapy from the list of "Differing Kinds of Therapies" (one that was not discussed in class) and write a brief description about it.

Group Activities

• Case Example Planning: Application of Cognitive-Behavioral interventions to working with a depressed client

Provide the class with a case study of a depressed individual and identify five nursing diagnoses (one–five). (Suggestion: Use a case example from Chapter 13.) Have the students count off in sequence in fives and regroup according to the number (all of the ones gather together, all of the twos gather, etc.). Assign each numerical group to develop some nursing interventions for their nursing diagnosis (one–five) using a cognitive-behavioral approach.

• Discussion: The future of individual therapy

Use the reflective thinking questions with this topic to stimulate class discussion.

Clinical Activities

• In the clinical area, interview the psychiatrist asking about her perspective on individual psychotherapy and which framework she prefers.

• Interview a nurse psychotherapist and ask about his perspective on individual psychotherapy and which framework he prefers.

Internet Activities

• Information on group therapy can be found on the home page for the American Group Psychotherapy Association:

http://www.agpa.org

• Descriptions of treatment for delusional disorders, including individual psychotherapy, are described on:

http://www.mentalhealth.com/rx/p23-ps02.html

NOTES

Family Therapy

Chapter
28

Competencies

Upon completion of this chapter, the learner will be able to:

1. Define different nursing approaches to working with the family.
2. Apply the concepts of family development and family life cycle to assessments in families.
3. Describe Bowen's family theory, and make an assessment of family level of differentiation.
4. Explain structural-family theory, and describe the nurse-therapist's role of entering into the family interactions and structure.
5. Use communications theory and the techniques of therapeutic communication to assist families in improving interfamilial communication.
6. Use the NANDA taxonomy to document family nursing diagnoses.
7. Complete family assessments using nursing assessment tools.
8. Use the nursing process to establish a plan of care for families in the psychiatric mental health setting.

Key Terms

Circular communication
Differentiation
Ecomap
Emotional cutoff
Family
Family attachment diagram
Family projection process
Genogram
Interventive questions
Multigenerational transmission process
Nuclear family emotional system
Power
Relativistic thinking
Sibling position
Societal regression
Triangulation

Teaching Methods and Strategies

Because there are numerous definitions of family, it is important to define the word *family* in a manner that allows students to understand the application of theoretical approaches to family therapy. The authors have defined family as *a social system composed of two or more persons who coexist within the context of some expectations of reciprocal affection, mutual responsibility, and temporal duration.* Students tend to have egocentric descriptions of what makes a family and discussing these can be quite revealing.

As mentioned in the chapters on individual and group therapies, the student as a beginning generalist nurse will not be performing the therapy. She may be involved in or observe the process of therapy facilitated by someone with advanced education and training. None the less, the student should have an understanding of the different approaches to providing family therapy.

Because most nurses do have a working understanding of the ideal of family development across the life cycle, the educator may wish to start with this content before moving on to the frameworks for therapy. In so doing, parallels can be drawn so that the student can begin to integrate the different concepts and approaches to caring for families.

Lesson Plans

Topic: Family Therapy

Competency 28.1

Define different nursing approaches to working with the family.

CONTENT OUTLINE

- Describe the family as context.
- Describe the family as client.
- Describe the family as a system.
- Describe the family as a component of society.

METHOD

Lecture
Slide/transparency
Review Figure 28-1
Review Table 28-1

Competency 28.2

Apply the concepts of family development and family life cycle to assessments in families.

CONTENT OUTLINE

- Describe family developmental theory as involving seven chronological stages:
  - Beginning family
  - Childbearing family
  - Family with preschool children

Family with teenagers
Family launching young adults
Family with middle-aged parents
Family in retirement

- Describe the life-cycle model of family patterns:
  - Traditional married couple with children
  - Divorced or post-divorce family
  - Remarried couple with children

METHOD

Lecture
Slide/transparency
Review Table 28-2

Competency 28.3

Describe Bowen's family theory, and make an assessment of family level of differentiation.

CONTENT OUTLINE

- Describe the view of the family in a multigenerational system context of patterns that repeat themselves.
- Identify the eight interwoven concepts of family systems theory:
  - Differentiation
  - Triangulation
  - Family projection process
  - Multigenerational transmission process
  - Nuclear family emotional system
  - Sibling position
  - Emotional cut-off
  - Societal regression
- Discuss the family dynamics/patterns at different levels of differentiation.

METHOD

Lecture
Review Table 28-3

Competency 28.4

Explain structural-family theory, and describe the nurse-therapist's role of entering into the family interactions and structure.

CONTENT OUTLINE

- Discuss the notion of the family system containing underlying organization, structures, roles, and functions to maintain equilibrium.
- Describe system constraints:
  - *Generic system:* Rules governing family organization, position, and power
  - *Idiosyncratic system:* Mutual expectations of family members
- Identify family subsystems formed according to:
  - *Generation:* Parent/children/grandparent
  - *Sex:* Male/female
  - *Interest:* Shared interests
  - *Function:* Who does what

METHOD

Lecture

Competency 28.5

Use communications theory and the techniques of therapeutic communication to assist families in improving interfamilial communication.

CONTENT OUTLINE

- Describe the goal of Satir's approaches to family communication.
- Describe Watzlawick's axioms about communication:
  - All behavior is communicated and conveys a message
  - All communication defines a relationship
  - Persons communicate both verbally and nonverbally
  - All communication is either symmetrical or complementary
- Describe nursing interactions based on communication theory.

METHOD

Lecture

Competency 28.6

Use the NANDA taxonomy to document family nursing diagnoses.

CONTENT OUTLINE

- Describe nursing diagnoses related to family processes.
- Describe nursing diagnoses related to family coping.
- Describe nursing diagnoses related to family home maintenance management.

METHOD

Lecture

Competency 28.7

Complete family assessments using nursing assessment tools.

CONTENT OUTLINE

- Demonstrate the use of the genogram and the ecomap in illustrating information assessed about a family.
- Assess the family structure:
  - Internal structure
  - External structure
  - Context
- Assess the family development/life cycle:
  - Stages
  - Tasks
  - Attachments

- Assess family function:

Instrumental	Expressive
Affective	Health care

METHOD

Discussion
Slide/transparency
Case example
Review Tables 28-3 and 28-4

Competency 27.8

Use the nursing process to establish a plan of care for families in the psychiatric mental health setting.

CONTENT OUTLINE

- Apply the nursing assessment to a case example.
- Apply the genogram information to the case example.
- Identify appropriate nursing diagnoses for the case example.
- Identify nursing actions to implement care based on nursing roles.

METHOD

Discussion
Slide/transparency
Case example
Review Tables 28-5 and 28-7

Learning Experiences

Theory Application

- Describe in more detail Satir's conjoint family therapy and the roles members play in family interactions.
- Review in-depth Minuchin's perspective on family subgroups and the relationships between subgroups.

Individual Activities

- In their journals, have students reflect on how they have experienced being a member of a family and then, using the systems theory, write about an experience of triangulation.
- Ask students to draw a three-generation genogram for their family, and identify their family's stage of development and state examples/supporting rationale.

Group Activities

- Discussion: As a class, review the case study care plan presented in this chapter.
- Application: Provide the class with another case example (suggest taking a case from Chapter 25, Survivors of Violence or Abuse). Proceed with the assessment, diagramming, and planning of care for the family.

Clinical Activities

- Use a genogram to diagram assessment information about family patterns for a client in your care.
- Discuss with the staff how (if) family therapy is utilized at the facility and who provides the therapy.

Internet Activities

- Periodicals and training materials can be accessed on the website for the Family Therapy Network:

  http://www.familytherapynetwork.com

- Information about the Ackerman Institute for the Family and its clinical training program in systemic family therapy can be accessed via:

  http://www.ackerman.org

NOTES

Group Therapy

Chapter 29

Competencies

Upon completion of this chapter, the learner will be able to:

1. Outline the three phases of group work: orientation phase, working phase, and termination phase.
2. Explain the terms *group dynamics, group content,* and *group process.*
3. Analyze the dynamics of a group session.
4. Define nursing roles with groups in the psychiatric mental health nursing setting.
5. Explain major theoretical approaches used in group therapy.
6. Explain the nursing role in supportive groups.
7. Compare and contrast different types of groups (socialization, recreation, educational, reality orientation, reminiscence, and self-help) in terms of purpose, nursing interventions, and evaluation.

Key Terms

Closed group	Group process
Group	Open group
Group content	Self-help group
Group dynamics	Supportive group
Group leader/facilitator	Therapy group

Teaching Methods and Strategies

Nurses are often called upon to work with groups of clients. The role of the nurse varies with the nurse's expertise and the purpose of the group. A nurse with knowledge of group process and group dynamics can increase the effectiveness of nursing care with many clients.

The nurse generalist is best prepared to assist in supportive groups where clients come together for the purposes of offering support, education, and/or socialization. The advanced practice psychiatric mental health nurse might also be called on to provide group therapy. Whether in the role of therapist, leader, or facilitator, it is important to understand the operations of groups

Lesson Plans

Topic: Group Therapy

Competency 29.1

Outline the three phases of group work: orientation phase, working phase, and termination phase.

CONTENT OUTLINE

- Describe the elements and dynamics of the orientation phase of a group.
- Describe the elements and dynamics of the working phase of a group.
- Describe the elements and dynamics of the termination phase of a group.

METHOD

Lecture
Slide/transparency
Review Table 29-1

Competency 29.2

Explain the terms *group dynamics, group content,* and *group process.*

CONTENT OUTLINE

- Define the term *group dynamics* as the underlying forces that work to produce behavior patterns within a group.
- Define *group content* as the specific topics, problems, or conditions addressed by the group as a whole.
- Define *group process* as the verbal and nonverbal interactions between group members.

METHOD

Lecture

Competency 29.3

Analyze the dynamics of a group session.

CONTENT OUTLINE

- Describe the dynamics of the group and its process with a group process diagram.
- Identify the elements of a group process diagram:
  - Members
  - Seating
  - Direction of verbal interactions
  - Nonverbal behaviors
  - Content and theme

- Identify roles that members may take in a group:

Problem solver	Naysayer
Controller	Supporter
Talker	Intimidator
Silent one	Devil's advocate

METHOD

Lecture
Slide/transparency
Review boxed information

Competency 29.4

Define nursing roles with groups in the psychiatric mental health nursing setting.

CONTENT OUTLINE

- Review the different roles of the nurse according to the ANA Scope of Practice statement.
- Discuss the roles of the nurse in groups.

METHOD

Lecture
Discussion
Slide/transparency
Review Table 29-2

Competency 29.5

Explain major theoretical approaches used in group therapy.

CONTENT OUTLINE

- Describe the psychoanalytic approach to group therapy.
- Describe the interpersonal approach to group therapy.
- Describe the existential approach to group therapy.
- Describe the cognitive-behavioral approach to group therapy.
- Describe psychodrama as a group therapy.

METHOD

Lecture
Slide/transparency

Competency 29.6

Explain the nursing role in supportive groups.

CONTENT OUTLINE

- Discuss the nurse's role as facilitator.
- Discuss the nurse's role of modeling appropriate behavior.
- Discuss the nurse's role in assisting in problem solving.

METHOD

Discussion

Competency 29.7

Compare and contrast different types of groups (socialization, recreational, educational, reality orientation, reminiscence, and self-help) in terms of purpose, nursing interventions, and evaluation.

CONTENT OUTLINE

- Describe the purpose, nursing interventions, and evaluation of a socialization group.
- Describe the purpose, nursing interventions, and evaluation of a recreational group.
- Describe the purpose, nursing interventions, and evaluation of an educational group.
- Describe the purpose, nursing interventions, and evaluation of a reality orientation group.
- Describe the purpose, nursing interventions, and evaluation of a reminiscence group.
- Describe the purpose, nursing interventions, and evaluation of a self-help group.

METHOD

Lecture
Discussion
Slide/transparency

Learning Experiences

Theory Application

- As the focus of a clinical conference, require students to do group process diagrams of the interactions of the clinical group, applying the theoretical information.
- Review the characteristics of effective group leaders.

Individual Activities

- The next time students attend a community meeting, for example, the League of Women Voters or a student organization meeting, have them examine their roles in the meeting.
- Encourage students to attend a self-help group meeting and then analyze the group process.

Group Activities

- Seminar: Divide the students into six groups. Assign each group to develop an 8-minute presentation about one of the supportive groups in which they identify the purpose, nurse's role, and some examples.
- Discussion: Psychoeducation groups: How are they most useful?

Clinical Activities

- Lead an educational group about coping with stress.

• Identify who "leads" which type of groups on the clinical unit (or at the agency).

Internet Activities

• General information about group therapy for the public and professionals can be found at this site provided by the Group Psychotherapy Association of Southern California:

http://www.gpasc.org.

• An example of a course that is offered in group psychotherapy is listed at this URL for the Applied Psychology Department at Antioch:

http://sparc.antiochne.edu/academics/courses/appsy-A1.html

NOTES

Community Mental Health Nursing

Chapter 30

Competencies

Upon completion of this chapter, the learner will be able to:

1. Describe the changing focus of care in the field of mental health.
2. Explain a conceptual framework for nursing practice with aggregates (population groups).
3. Explain selected strategies that can be used to improve the health status of aggregates (population groups).
4. Describe nursing practice with aggregates (population groups).

Key Terms

Aggregate	Population
Capitation	Primary prevention
Case management	Program for assertive community treatment (PACT)
Community health nursing	Prospective payment system
Community mental health	Public health nursing
Community support system (CSS)	Secondary prevention
Deinstitutionalization	Tertiary prevention
Home health nursing	
Managed care	

Teaching Methods and Strategies

The trend to provide more care in the community continues. The role of the psychiatric mental health nurse in the community is simultaneously evolving. During this time of change, there may be community confusion about how the nurse can implement community-focused care.

The educator has the role of explaining the larger focus of aggregate care and assisting students to implement the strategies that support this focus. There may be opportunities for community-based clinical experiences where students can begin to practice these roles. With faculty guidance, they can experience this re-emerging dimension of psychiatric mental health nursing.

Lesson Plans

Topic: Community Mental Health Nursing

Competency 30.1

Describe the changing focus of care in the field of mental health.

CONTENT OUTLINE

- Describe the historical factors that led to the community focus for care of the mental patient.
- Describe legislative factors that led to the focus of community mental health.
- Describe economic factors that influence the shift to community-based care.
- Describe the features of PACT services.

METHOD

Lecture
Review boxed information: Description of PACT Services

Competency 30.2

Explain a conceptual framework for nursing practice with aggregates (population groups).

CONTENT OUTLINE

- Define aggregate as a population or defined group.
- Describe how aggregate data are used to identify needs. Plan services and evaluate programs in the community.
- Describe different aggregate-focused frameworks:
  - Client-centered model
  - Case management model
  - Capitation and managed-care models
  - Public health model

METHOD

Lecture
Review Figure 30-2

Competency 30.3

Explain selected strategies that can be used to improve the health status of aggregates (population groups).

CONTENT OUTLINE

- Describe the strategy of epidemiological studies.
- Describe the public health model of needs assessment and priority determination for high-risk aggregates.
- Discuss the role of nurses in public health care.

METHOD

Lecture
Discussion

Competency 30.4

Describe nursing practice with aggregates (population groups).

CONTENT OUTLINE

- Describe primary prevention nursing strategies:
  - Teaching classes on stress management
  - Conducting support groups of children in transition
  - Teaching parenting skills
  - Health fair educational information
  - Data collection for local needs assessment
- Describe secondary prevention nursing strategies:
  - Staffing crisis centers
  - Involvement on rape counseling team
  - Operating shelter for abused women
  - Screening clients with debilitating chronic disease for mental health problems (e.g., depression)
- Describe tertiary prevention nursing strategies:
  - Teaching socialization skills to those in psychosocial or partial hospitalization programs
  - Monitoring effectiveness of aftercare services with follow-up appointments
  - Conducting medication management groups for those in half-way/transitional housing

METHOD

Lecture
Discussion
Slide/transparency

Learning Experiences

Theory Application

- Review the public health model of prevention and the nursing foci at each level of care.
- Review the *Healthy People 2000* report of aggregate needs related to mental health.

Individual Activities

- In their journals, ask students to reflect on their perspective about how community-based care and individual care differ.
- Have students identify which aggregate framework is being used in the practice of their primary health care provider.

Group Activities

- Discussion: As a class, review the PACT services and discuss the reflective thinking questions.
- Discussion: As a group, discuss the components of a community support system. Use Figure 30-2 as a basis for the discussion.

Clinical Activities

- Create a resource board in the clinical area with the information about the National Alliance for the Mentally Ill (NAMI) and local support groups such as DRADA (Depression and Related Affective Disorders Association).
- Spend time at a community-based agency and discuss with the nurse the aggregate focus as it is implemented at the agency.

Internet Activities

- The University of Pennsylvania has multiple links for community mental health projects and services for special populations at its Home Nursing Agency web site. Included is information about rural nursing centers that provide outreach for the medically underserved populations and housing for the homeless mentally ill:

  http://www.hhdev.psu.edu/nurs/rncp.htm

- The Department of Psychosocial and Community Health of the University of Washington School of Nursing is involved in numerous community mental health projects:

  http://www.son.washington.edu/departments/pch

Complementary and Somatic Therapies

Chapter 31

Competencies

Upon completion of this chapter, the learner will be able to:

1. Describe the use of six complementary modalities as nursing interventions in psychiatric mental health care.
2. Intervene to control escalating anger in a client.
3. Describe the use of physical restraints and seclusion in control of violent behavior.
4. Describe the use of light therapy for treatment of seasonal affective disorder (SAD).
5. Describe the current indications for electroconvulsive therapy (ECT), and provide nursing care to a client undergoing the procedure.

Key Terms

Anger control assistance	Light therapy (phototherapy)
Animal-assisted therapy	Massage
Complementary modalities	Music therapy
Electroconvulsive therapy (ECT)	Relaxation
Energy-based modalities	Seclusion
Guided imagery	Somatic therapies
Healing touch	Therapeutic imagery
Hypnosis	Therapeutic massage
	Therapeutic touch (TT)

Teaching Methods and Strategies

There are many alternative and complementary strategies used to deal with stress and emotional disturbances. No doubt, many students are familiar with many of these alternatives. So are clients, many of whom spend a great deal of money on supplements and devices to "help deal with their problems." As an educator, it is important to assist the student to develop an objective understanding of these modalities.

Lesson Plans

Topic: Complementary and Somatic Therapy

Competency 31.1

Describe the use of six complementary modalities as nursing interventions in psychiatric mental health care.

CONTENT OUTLINE

- Describe the use of relaxation and guided mental imagery in psychiatric mental health nursing care.
- Describe the use of hypnosis in psychiatric mental health nursing care.
- Describe the use of massage in psychiatric mental health nursing care.
- Describe the use of energy-based modalities (therapeutic touch and healing touch) in psychiatric mental health nursing care.
- Describe the use of music therapy in psychiatric mental health nursing care.
- Describe the use of animal-assisted therapy in psychiatric mental health nursing care.

METHOD

Lecture
Slide/transparency
Review Table 31-1

Competency 31.2

Intervene to control escalating anger in a client.

CONTENT OUTLINE

- Discuss the nurse's role of intervening in controlling anger in a client.
- Review assessment for risk of violence.
- Describe the techniques used in anger control:
  - Limit access to frustrating situations
  - Provide physical outlets, large muscle activities
  - Use a journal
  - Ensure adequate personal space
  - Decrease environmental stimuli

METHOD

Discussion

Competency 31.3

Describe the use of physical restraints and seclusion in control of violent behavior.

CONTENT OUTLINE

- Describe the guidelines for use of physical restraints.
- Describe the appropriate application of physical restraint devices.

- Describe what to observe while the client is in restraints.
- Describe the seclusion process.
- Describe the procedural elements of use of seclusion.

METHOD

Lecture

Competency 31.4

Describe the use of light therapy for treatment of Seasonal Affective Disorder (SAD).

CONTENT OUTLINE

- Define phototherapy as the use of therapeutic lighting in the treatment of individuals with Seasonal Affective Disorder.
- Describe what is involved in light therapy.
- Identify the nurse's role in phototherapy.

METHOD

Lecture

Competency 31.5

Describe the current indications for electroconvulsive therapy (ECT), and provide nursing care to a client undergoing the procedure.

CONTENT OUTLINE

- Define electroconvulsive therapy.
- Identify the uses of ECT as a somatic therapy to treat mental illness.
- Review the nurse's role and nursing care of clients undergoing ECT procedure.

METHOD

Lecture

Learning Experiences

Theory Application

- Review the specific uses of ECT as well as unipolar and bipolar electrode placement.
- Review the therapeutic uses of acupuncture in the treatment of mental disorders.

Individual Activities

- Have students review the list of complementary approaches, select one approach, and find three articles about its use for emotional/mental disorders.
- Encourage students to contact a spokesperson for "Pets-on-Wheels," then write about their reactions to the experiences in their journals.

Group Activities

- Discussion: What are some of the potential risks and "cautions" about use of massage for treatment of emotional disorders?
- Panel: Complementary practitioners

  Arrange for a panel of practitioners to discuss their approaches to treatment of mental illness. Then, using one case example, ask each practitioner to discuss his approach.

Clinical Activities

- Review the procedures and guidelines for use of restraints in the clinical facility/agency.
- Ask staff to share an experience when client anger escalated and how the staff responded.

Internet Activities

- For a description about guided mental imagery and also some ideas for music, check this site:

  http://www.desertheartmusic.com/WhatisGIM.html
- A glossary with links to descriptions of complementary/alternative therapies can be found at:

  http://www.hml.org/CHIS/glossary.html

Unit

5

Caring for the Nurse

The last unit of this text is devoted to the nurse as the caregiver. To perform best in the demanding roles of the psychiatric mental health nurse, it is important to engage in activities that are restorative and protective of self.

Chapter 32 presents several self-care modalities. It focuses on the role of the nurse as a self-healer as well as on healthy professional development.

Chapter 33 is titled "Friday Night at the Movies." Often there are many educational elements in movies in addition to general entertainment. The authors have searched for movies that support the topics of each chapter in the first three units. Other movies that provide examples of therapeutic interventions have been listed to complement the content of Unit 4. A brief description of how each movie is linked to the content of the chapter or unit is provided. The use of movies as an educational tool varies greatly. Some suggested activities have been provided. However, there are many other ways to utilize this medium for educational purposes.

NOTES

Self-Care Modalities

Chapter 32

Competencies

Upon completion of this chapter, the learner will be able to:

1. Define meditation, imagery, and self-hypnosis.
2. Describe the differences among these three self-help modalities.
3. Explain the importance of self-help for psychiatric caregivers.
4. Describe a few means by which support groups can be developed.
5. Identify three ways in which humor promotes healing.
6. Employ the use of relaxation and imagery for self-care.
7. Identify two reasons for centering prior to entering a psychiatric care unit.
8. Use the nursing self-care process to achieve a higher level of professional wellness as a caregiver.

Key Terms

Burnout
Circadian rhythm
Parasympathetic system response
Sympathetic system response
Victim consciousness

Teaching Methods and Strategies

The question of how to teach someone to take care of self generally presents a puzzle to nurses. As a profession, nurses tend to spend time caring for others and not caring for self. However, the healthier perspective is to strike a balance. The educator has a role as a model for students. Through interacting and talking with the educator and by observing the lived experience of balanced attitudes, behaviors, and practices, the student can learn much.

Lesson Plans

Topic: Self-Care Modalities

Competency 32.1

Define meditation, imagery, and self-hypnosis.

CONTENT OUTLINE

- Describe meditation for relaxation.
- Describe the practice of imagery.
- Describe self-hypnosis.

METHOD

Lecture
Slide/transparency

Competency 32.2

Describe the differences among these three self-help modalities.

CONTENT OUTLINE

- Describe how the approaches of meditation, imagery, and self-hypnosis are different from each other.
- Describe how the approaches of meditation, imagery, and self-hypnosis can be similar.

METHOD

Discussion

Competency 32.3

Explain the importance of self-help for psychiatric caregivers.

CONTENT OUTLINE

- Define burnout.
- Discuss the interwoven elements of attitudes, behavior, and practice.
- Define self-help.
- Describe internal self-assessment techniques.
- Describe the importance of self-help to healthy living.

METHOD

Lecture
Discussion

Competency 32.4

Describe a few means by which support groups can be developed.

CONTENT OUTLINE

- Discuss the strategy of active, intentional listening with an open heart.
- Discuss the role of offering suggestions.

METHOD

Discussion

Competency 32.5

Identify three ways in which humor promotes healing.

CONTENT OUTLINE

- Discuss the role of humor in relaxation.
- Discuss the role of humor as a coping strategy.
- Discuss the role of humor as a means of developing a greater sense of mastery.

METHOD

Discussion

Competency 32.6

Employ the use of relaxation and imagery for self-care.

CONTENT OUTLINE

- Demonstrate one relaxation exercise.
- Facilitate a group imagery exercise for the class.
- Discuss other ways to use relaxation and imagery in self-care.

METHOD

Discussion
Experiential exercise

Competency 32.7

Identify two reasons for centering prior to entering a psychiatric care unit.

CONTENT OUTLINE

- Describe the usefulness of centering for balancing internal energies.
- Discuss the importance of centering for clear thinking.
- Discuss the importance of centering to be better able to effectively and meaningfully relate to the client.

METHOD

Discussion

Competency 32.8

Use the nursing self-care process to achieve a higher level of professional wellness as a caregiver.

CONTENT OUTLINE

- Practice one nursing self-care process and describe how it has facilitated professional wellness.
- Discuss "stories" of enhanced professional wellness related to self-care processes.

METHOD

Discussion
Experiential exercise

Learning Experiences

Theory Application

- Review the theoretical basis for the use of humor in healing.
- Review the theoretical information about energy work.

Individual Activities

- For one week, have students practice the "Release Balloon Exercise" every day and record in their journals how they felt before, during, and after the exercise.
- Ask students their thoughts about energy balancing.

Group Activities

- Discussion: How do nurses use humor to cope with the stresses of the profession? Let's talk . . . laugh . . . cry . . . about it?
- Panel: Ask a group of psychiatric nurses to join in a discussion panel about the need for and strategies to facilitate the improvement of nurses' self-health and caring for the caregiver.

Clinical Activities

- Identify one strategy used by the nursing staff on the unit to promote self-care.
- With the staff, practice the "Release Balloon Exercise." Then discuss responses and ideas about the exercise.

Internet Activities

- Visit:
  http://www4.allencol.edu/~sey0/orem.html

Friday Night at the Movies

Chapter 33

Competencies

Upon completion of this chapter, the learner will be able to:

1. Recognize that learning is possible in many situations.

Teaching Methods and Strategies

This chapter "speaks for itself" when it comes to teaching strategies. As mentioned in the overview for Unit 5, integrating the use of videos as a medium for learning has long been a tradition in nursing. Through use of "generic" movies, the importance of psychiatric nursing can be highlighted. Movies provide the educator with case examples, with examples for application of concepts, with support for the need for mental health care, and on occasion, with role enactment. Movies can be used as a focus of classroom teaching or clinical conferences. One strategy is to use movies at the end of a course in psychiatric mental health nursing to excite the students with just how much they have learned. Of course, they may never look at a movie in quite the same way again. Upon completion of the course in psychiatric mental health nursing, they will never look at nursing in quite the same way again either.

Lesson Plans

Topic: Films

Competency 33.1

Recognize that learning is possible in many situations.

CONTENT OUTLINE

- Watch a move about a mental disorder.
- Watch a movie about a special population.
- Watch a movie about a treatment modality.

METHOD

Discussion
Video

Learning Experiences

Theory Application

- Show the movie *Through a Glass Darkly* to emphasize the behaviors noted in schizophrenia.

Individual Activities

- Have students watch the movie *Sybil* and then in their journals, write their reactions to what it must be like for someone having multiple personality disorder.

Group Activities

- As a class, watch the first fifteen minutes of *Prince of Tides* and discuss what family dynamics have been displayed.

Clinical Activities

- As part of a planned activity with a group of clients who are recovering from substance abuse, watch the movie *Postcards from the Edge.* Ask them to discuss the movie afterwards in terms of their own experiences and recovery.

NOTES